SATTVIK
COOKING

Also by the author

Yoga for All
The 12 Yogic Principles for Making Marriages Work

SATTVIK COOKING

Modern Avatars of
VEDIC FOODS

HANSAJI J. YOGENDRA

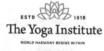
ESTD 1918
The Yoga Institute
WORLD HARMONY BEGINS WITHIN

RUPA

Published by
Rupa Publications India Pvt. Ltd 2021
7/16, Ansari Road, Daryaganj
New Delhi 110002

Sales centres:
Allahabad Bengaluru Chennai
Hyderabad Jaipur Kathmandu
Kolkata Mumbai

ISBN: 978-93-90918-85-0

Fifth impression 2022

10 9 8 7 6 5

The moral right of the author has been asserted.

Printed in India

CONTENTS

FOREWORD

In my years of cooking and understanding food, there's a lot that has touched me and much more that I am still becoming aware of. Over a period of time, food has become my window to cultures, people and world as seen and experienced. At some point in time when my spiritual and culinary journeys merged I realized that we are all made of food 'Ann Purna Brahma'. Our thoughts, our aspirations, our emotions are all food.

I have realized with enough proof that happy people make happy food, and not just that, food made by happy people makes the person who's eating it happy as well. Food transfers intent and emotions—mothers cooking being a case in the point.

It doesn't stop here, happy ingredients which have grown sustainably and without stress, external push or manipulation (read seasonal, chemical and fertilizer free Ingredients) make for dishes that bring Real happiness to the mind, body and the soul. A happiness that's not only sustainable because it's in sync with our basic nature and the basic nature of our relationship with our surroundings and seasons, but also infectious enough to wirelessly spread at raging speeds.

I have been blessed to know Hansaji for over three years and can truly endorse the fact that she embodies this happiness. Besides the innumerable recognitions and awards, her smile is proof enough that she has cracked the code of 'happy food', that creates sustainable happiness for the mind, body and soul.

The food and the approach to food at The Yoga Institute is a small peak into her happiness universe or may I say her 'recipe of happiness'.

I am sure this book, through its food philosophy and its recipes, will connect you to yourself because that is the only and ultimate objective of food, touching all our senses to experience and hold onto real joy.

Ranveer Brar
11 May 2021

INTRODUCTION

The book provides an in-depth perspective on diet in Ayurveda and yogic Sattvik ahar, and their significance with respect to modern evidence-based nutrition.

Yoga, the sister science of Ayurveda, aims at personal transformation through holistic healing. It considers food to be much more than mere fuel for the body. Food affects all the koshas (sheaths/layers) of the body. The grossest sheath of the body is called the Annamaya Kosha, as it is nourished by food and grows from it. However, food also extends its effect on other entities of our existence such as energy, mind, intellect, emotions and soul.

"Susnigdhamadhuraahaaraschachaturthanshavivarjitah
Bhujyate shivasamprityeh mithaarah saa uchyate"

(Hathapradipika-1/58)

These lines are part of classical yogic literature and translate to mean: sweet food is that which is pleasant tasting, satvik, easy-to-digest and fresh. Such food is called mitahara. It is not necessarily high in sugar. One must consume it in moderation, leaving one-fourth of the stomach empty as an offering to the Lord.

The book also reviews eating as per the ayurvedic clock and calendar, laying emphasis on ritucharya or seasonal recommendations on diet and lifestyle, and dincharya or the disciplined daily routine.

In a bid to reach out to millennials, this book decodes traditional Vedic eating with a deep dive into shadrasas, or the six tastes and their effect on our body. The book also discusses jnanendriya or experiencing food through senses.

As you traverse through this rich treasure of culinary delights from different parts of India and across the world, you will find delectable recipes modified to conform to yogic concepts.

The kitchen pharmacy and ancient superfoods will empower the reader to translate kitchen ingredients into powerful natural remedies that are scientifically backed by research. Our immunity-boosting decoctions, brews, ayurvedic kadhas and ukkalas are a brilliant combination of high dose of virtuous herbs and spices present in our kitchen.

In the intelligent snack section, the book aims to satisfy the palates of all age groups. The international and fusion snacks mentioned in the book are a unique blend of taste and health for millennials. Every recipe is unique with functional foods and curated to provide naturally high antioxidant and anti-inflammatory properties, with immense health benefits.

Each recipe comes with a description of its ingredients and nutritive value, an advisory on serving portions, and cooking skills. Most recipes in the book are simple and nutritious.

Health watchers and fitness enthusiasts will find the book useful as every recipe comes with a 'know your nutrition' section, which is a description of varied nutrients, enabling users to understand and appreciate the goodness of food. In addition, the book suggests smart cooking tips with the recipe.

In today's digital era, recipes count their major macronutrients, such as carbohydrates, proteins, fats, fiber, and other micronutrients of high health significance like sodium, potassium, calcium, iron and omega 3.

Healthy food on the move contains tantalizing recipes on travel. It is also perfect for school tiffins and snack breaks at the office.

Whilst understanding taste is prime, the section on chutneys, a dollop of happiness, is a unique salt-reducing effort with the inclusion of various functional foods (or foods that can also work as medicine).

Modern medical science lays great emphasis on gut health. The gut is also called the 'second brain'. This can be easily correlated to Ayurveda's belief that the root cause of all disease is poor gut health. Readers can appreciate good probiotic and prebiotic recipes, which can soothe the gut, keeping it happy and healthy.

Understanding the mind-body connection is the utmost goal of the Sattvik diet.

Food and mood are completely interlinked, and modern-day stress can completely disrupt eating patterns by inducing emotional and stress eating. The book provides simple guidance to foods that can keep stress at bay and improve cognitive and mental health.

Jagrukta or mindful eating is the basic principle that every yoga aspirant should follow. Today, research completely endorses mindful eating as an effective tool for weight loss and binge-eating disorders. Through simple steps prescribed in the book one can gain mindfulness on a daily basis.

In the end, the book echoes that food is divinity. The Annabrahma significantly emphasizes the concept 'From the food we come, we grow and we become'. The concept of krutagyata lays emphasis on the attitude and gratitude of the eater.

Naaznin Husein
Editor and compiler

(Naaznin is a celebrity dietitian, counseling many Bollywood actors and sports celebrities. She is a qualified dietitian who combines holistic lifestyle management with evidence-based nutrition, fused with traditional Sattvik practices.)

1

REVIVING ANCIENT PRACTICES

AHAR: A VEDIC PERSPECTIVE ON DIET

'Life (ayu) is the combination (samyoga) of body, senses, mind and the reincarnating soul. Ayurveda is a more sacred science of life beneficial to humans both in this world and world beyond.'

—Charaka

The term 'ayurveda' comes from two Sanskrit words—*ayus* and *veda*, which translate to mean 'life' and 'knowledge'. *Anna* (food) and *ahaar* (diet) form the central pillars of this science of life. According to Ayurveda, both health and illness emerge from the food we consume. It emphasizes the holistic and personalized nature of the treatment. The comprehensive principles of Ayurveda stand on the strong foundation of philosophical texts, traditional knowledge and scientific evidence.

Ayurveda's individualistic approach functions on the concept of *tridoshas* (the three life forces)—which make up the body constitution. Of course, it is different for each person. Identifying your dominant *dosha* and adopting dietary and lifestyle changes to pacify it forms the basis of Ayurvedic treatment.

A QUICK GUIDE TO DOSHAS

What are doshas?

Doshas are body humours that govern the various physical processes that occur in the body. They are born from the *panchamahabhutas* (the five cosmic elements).

- Air and ether form *vata*
- Fire and water form *pitta*
- Earth and water form *kapha*

How does vata work in our bodies?

Vata, in its balanced state, is responsible for movement. It facilitates respiration, preserving sensory activity and sending brain impulses. When vitiated, it leads to dryness of skin and lips, fatigue, disturbed menstrual cycle, weakened sensory response, cracking joints, insomnia and constipation.

What can I do to pacify vata?

- Choose sweet, sour, or salty foods as they bring vata under control
- Include more of wheat and gram flour products, cooked apples, watermelon, milk and milk products, carrots, tomatoes, beetroot, sweet potatoes, nuts, figs, dates, quinoa, brown rice, green gram, ghee, sesame oil, olive oil, carom seeds, turmeric, cumin, black pepper and sugarcane in your diet
- Massage regularly using sesame oil

How does pitta work in our bodies?

Pitta in its balanced state oversees digestion, preserves the skin's smoothness and lustre, facilitates hunger and thirst signals, maintains the vision, and preserves heat in the body. However when disturbed, pitta may lead to hair loss, burning sensations, sensitivity to light, intense hunger and thirst, oily skin and scalp, as well as yellow discoloration of eyes and skin.

What can I do to pacify pitta?

- Have food that is bitter, astringent and sweet
- Plan easily digestible meals that include green gram, apricots, coconut, papaya, bell peppers, cauliflower, sprouts, cucumber, leafy vegetables, amaranth, oats, lentils, chickpeas, ghee, almonds, pumpkin seeds, honey, coconut oil, olive oil, Indian gooseberry, saffron, mint, ginger, cinnamon and rice
- Do not sleep during the day

How does kapha work in our bodies?

In its balanced state, kapha maintains firmness and stability in the body, lubricates joints, and invokes feelings of peace and love. When aggravated, it builds excessive phlegm and blocks the sinuses, causes headaches, decreases the digestive capacity, increases cravings for salty foods and sometimes causes breathlessness.

What can I do to pacify kapha?

- Include barley, berries, pomegranate, lemon, mango, broccoli, spinach, carrots, millets, quinoa, honey, chickpeas, flaxseeds, asafoetida, paprika, ginger, garlic, fennel, cardamom, olive oil, ghee and other easily digestible foods in your diet
- Rise before sunrise and start your day with some energizing exercises such as *surya namaskar*
- Sip warm tea made with ginger or spices and herbs such as fennel, coriander, basil, cardamom or saffron

SCIENCE MEETS ANCIENT WISDOM

Researchers have marveled at the parallelism found between the Freudian theories and Lewinian models of psychology and the classical Indian philosophy of *Samkhya*. Here's how ayurvedic concepts correspond to modern psychological findings.

Concept	Ancient ayurvedic science	Modern medical evidence
Doshas meet Hippocrates 'Humors'	• Vata (air) • Pitta (bile) • Kapha (phlegm) • Rakta (blood)	• Melancholic (excess spleen) • Choleric (excess bile) • Sanguine (excess blood) • Phlegmatic (excess phlegm)
Purusha and prakriti meet personality	• Purusha (the spirit) • Prakriti (the material world) Goal: The highest state of knowledge is to realize that one is Purusha	• German poet Goethe described personality as 'the supreme value' • Philosopher Immanuel Kant believed that self realization helped in the development of human personality
Vasanas meet Freud's Id	Vasana is described as the unmanifested factor, which is a result of all human experiences	Freud described Id as the unconscious self, the seat of our wishes, desires and pleasure-seeking activities
Panchamahabhutas meet Cosmogony	Panchamahabhutas are the five cosmic elements namely—prithvi (earth), vayu (air), agni (fire), jala (water) and akash (space). These make up the entire universe.	In 450 BC, Empedocles doctrine on cosmogony highlighted four cosmic elements—air, earth, fire, and water.

Yoga, the sister science of ayurveda, too aims at personal transformation through holistic healing. It considers food to be much more than mere fuel for the body. Food affects all the *koshas* (sheaths/layers) of the body. The grossest sheath of the body is rightly called the *annamaya kosha*, as it is nourished by food and grows from it. However, food also extends its effect on other entities of our existence such as energy, mind, intellect, emotions and soul.

> *'Susnigdhamadhuraahaaraschachaturthanshavivarjitah*
> *Bhujyate shivasamprityeh mithaarah saa uchyate'*

(Hathapradipika-1/58)

The above lines belong to a classical yogic literature and translate to mean—Sattvik food, which is pleasant tasting, easy-to-digest, and fresh is called *mitahara*. One must consume it in moderation, leaving one-fourth of the stomach empty as an offering to Lord Shiva.

THE BIRTH OF AYURVEDA

Ayurveda, the oldest healing science, has an interesting story of origin. According to Indian mythological texts, this is how the divine science was passed on:

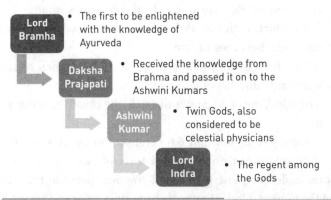

Lord Bramha
• The first to be enlightened with the knowledge of Ayurveda

Daksha Prajapati
• Received the knowledge from Brahma and passed it on to the Ashwini Kumars

Ashwini Kumar
• Twin Gods, also considered to be celestial physicians

Lord Indra
• The regent among the Gods

Lord Indra graced three sages who meditated intensely to end the human suffering and diseases with the wisdom of three different specialties.

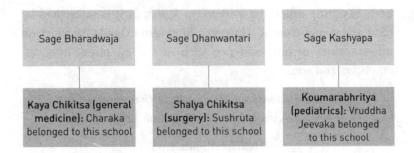

Sage Bharadwaja	Sage Dhanwantari	Sage Kashyapa
Kaya Chikitsa (general medicine): Charaka belonged to this school	Shalya Chikitsa (surgery): Sushruta belonged to this school	Koumarabhritya (pediatrics): Vruddha Jeevaka belonged to this school

Ayurveda and yoga advise against overeating and urge individuals to eat food with the awareness that they are making an offering to the supreme inner consciousness, and not simply to gratify their senses.

Trigunas: You Become What You Eat

INTRODUCTION TO SATTVIK AHAR

'That which is the subtle portion of curds, when churned, rises upwards and becomes butter.

In the same manner, my child, the subtle portion of the earth (food), when eaten, rises upwards and becomes mind.

That which is the subtle portion of water, when drunk, rises upwards and becomes breath.

That which is the subtle portion of the fire, when consumed, rises upwards and becomes speech.

For mind, my child comes of earth, the breath of water, speech of fire.'

Chandogya Upanishad 6.6 (Translation by Max Muller)

Ancient Indian philosophical texts of *Samkhya* believe that subtle underlying energies called *trigunas* pervade the universe and the human mind. They are called sattva, rajas and tamas. Sattva is pure, energizing, vitalizing and light. Rajas are stimulating, passionate, ambitious and domineering. And tamas is dull, inactive, heavy and impure.

The *trigunas* permeate our body and mind through food. Food has an inherent quality. In *Chanakya Shatakam*, the philosopher Chanakya states that 'just like the lamp feeds on darkness and produces soot, man too generates what he consumes'. Sattvik food enriches the soul and energizes the body and mind. They create purity, virtue, serenity and happiness. Rajasic food keeps one bound to passions and primal instincts. It leads to pain, jealousy, aggression, delusion and attachment. And tamasic food can push one into ignorance, pessimism and laziness.

Sattvik food	Rajasic food	Tamasic food
• Milk and milk products • Rice • Pulses such as split red gram split, bengal gram and field beans • Sprouted beans • Fenugreek leaves • Pumpkin • Gourds • Honey • Jaggery • Fresh fruits and vegetables, especially custard apple, apple, pomegranate banana, fenugreek leaves, pumpkin, gourds, cucumber and lady's finger • Millets • Mild herbs and spices such as ginger, turmeric, coriander and cardamom • Ghee	• Fish[1] • Eggs • Goat, sheep and chicken meat • Wine • Beer • White sugar • Radish • Deep-fried food • Coffee and tea • Jam • Ice cream and chocolates	• Processed and preserved foods such as biscuits and wafers • Frozen and canned food such as pickles and sauces • Stale, rotten, reheated, leftover foods • Pork, beef and non-scaly fish meat • Strong brews and intoxicants • Strongly spiced and seasoned food • Garlic • Onion

[1]People residing in the coastal regions of India regard fish to be a fruit of the ocean and consider it Sattvik.

In chapter 17 of the *Bhagavad Gita*, Lord Krishna says,

> *ayuh-sattva-balarogya-*
> *sukha-priti-vivardhanah*
> *rasyah snigdhah sthira hrdya*
> *aharah Sattvika-priyah*
> *katv-amla-lavanaty-usna-*
> *tiksna-ruksa-vidahinah*
> *ahara rajasasyesta*
> *duhkha-sokamaya-pradah*
> *yata-yamam gata-rasam*
> *puti paryusitam ca yat*
> *ucchistam api camedhyam*
> *bhojanam tamasa-priyam*

This means:

Juicy, unctuous, sweet and pure food is considered Sattvik. This food is palatable and pleasing to the heart. Consuming them gives longevity, strength, satisfaction, happiness and health. Bitter, sour, salty, hot, pungent and dry food is considered rajasic. Excessive consumption of such food leads to sorrow and sickness. Stale, tasteless, putrid, decomposed and impure food is considered tamasic. It takes one towards ignorance.

Science Meets Ancient Wisdom

Research proves that the micronutrient concentration (especially beta carotene, vitamin C, riboflavin, thiamin, folic acid, zinc, copper and iron) and total dietary fibre is the highest in Sattvik food and lowest in tamasic food. Additionally, the overall fat content tends to be the highest in tamasic meals and lowest in Sattvik meals. Tamasic food is associated with increased levels of anxiety.

DID YOU KNOW?

A Historical Sneak-Peek into Ashramas and Eating Patterns: Every stage of life (or ashrama) had recommendations for different rules and dietary pattern.

- *Students who lived in their teachers' homes (for the first 25 years of their life):* Pleasure-stimulating foods such as honey, meat, spices, onion, garlic, acid dishes and others were believed to stimulate passions. On certain days, students were made to beg so that they understand the importance of food.
- *Householders (25 to 50 years):* Washing hands before and after eating and dining without talking was considered essential.
- Before eating, the householder had to offer some food to the Gods and then serve children, old men, newlywed girls, sick people and pregnant women. He should also set aside food for dogs, the marginalized, people who were ill, birds and insects.
- *During retirement (50 to 75 years):* They had to avoid cultivated grains and practice diet consisting predominantly of fruits. During fasts, bread and snacks were made of water chestnut or lotus seed flour instead of wheat, onion, turmeric, garlic, ginger. Urad dal was banned.
- *In the final stages of life (after 75 till death):* Eating early in the morning, late in the evening, or between meals or eating too much was avoided. Consumption of Sattvik ahar in small quantities was advised.

2

KNOW YOUR BODY:
THE AYURVEDA GUIDE

KOSHAS: THE MULTI-LAYERED HUMAN

Our body is the physical and material sheath of our existence. It is a complex system that consists of multiple layers. An in-depth understanding of this enables us to stay energetic and stress-free, and transform our health from the grassroots. The five *koshas* or layers that compose our personality are described in a yoga classic called the *Taittiriya Upanishad*.

Annamaya kosha

The first dimension or kosha is called *Annamaya kosha* or the physical body/sthula sharira. Anna means food, and the physical body, composed of flesh and bones, is made up of food and sustained by food. Food that keeps the Annamaya kosha healthy are fresh fruits and vegetables as well as freshly prepared meals. Consuming overcooked, stale food or meat reduces the vitality of the Annamaya kosha.

Pranamaya kosha

Pranamaya kosha is the second layer or sukshma sharira. Prana is the vital energy that keeps the body alive. Just as water poured in a vessel takes its shape, the pranamaya too fully occupies the Annamaya kosha. Prana remains the same, but performs different functions in different parts of the body and is, hence, termed differently. Regular pranayama practices replenish the vitality of Pranamaya kosha.

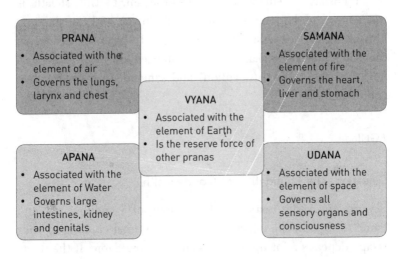

PRANA
- Associated with the element of air
- Governs the lungs, larynx and chest

SAMANA
- Associated with the element of fire
- Governs the heart, liver and stomach

VYANA
- Associated with the element of Earth
- Is the reserve force of other pranas

APANA
- Associated with the element of Water
- Governs large intestines, kidney and genitals

UDANA
- Associated with the element of space
- Governs all sensory organs and consciousness

Manomaya kosha

In Vedanta, the *Manomaya kosha* is referred to as the mind. It receives information from sensory organs and forms perceptions and thoughts. This sheath also deals with emotions. Anger, doubt, lust, delusion and depression—all arise from this kosha. Sattvik food keeps the Manomaya kosha healthy. Practising pratyahara (withdrawal of senses) and mudras keep the mind focused.

Vigyanamaya kosha

Vigyanamaya kosha is the seat of intellect. It is where our *viveka buddhi* (discerning power) resides. This is the centre of our thinking, sense of discrimination, and judgement. Together, the Manomaya and Vigyanamaya koshas make up the mind. A harmonious and supportive environment is essential for this kosha. Meditation, studying, reading and contemplation, along with a Sattvik diet, help revitalize the Vigyanamaya kosha.

Anandamaya kosha

Anandamaya kosha is the blissful sheath and the innermost of all koshas. It surrounds atman—the spirit. This sheath is the source of happiness, ecstasy, fulfillment and satisfaction. The sattva (brightness, illumination, purity balance) resides in the Anandamaya kosha, which is vitalized by three practices: Seva (service), bhakti (devotion) and samadhi (deep meditative contemplation).

AGNI

Digestion: The Foundation of Good Health

Several Ayurvedic texts use the analogy of a cooking pot and flame to explain the effect of agni. The optimal cooking of your recipe depends a lot upon the strength of the flame. If the flame is too low, the food may take longer to cook or may remain undercooked. If the flame is too high, the food may burn. Only when the flame is appropriately strong will the food be cooked evenly and to perfection. The same applies to the process of digestion. The cooking pot relates to our stomach, the flame to our agni and the cooking process to our digestion.

Identify your agni

If one feels activated and charged after meals, can digest food without discomfort, has a good immune system and a stable appetite, it can be said that the person has *Sama agni* (a balanced digestive fire).

If one feels lethargic and lazy after meals, has a low appetite, gains weight easily and has frequent episodes of indigestion, cough, vomiting, excessive saliva production and weakness, one may be suffering from *Manda agni* (a dull digestive fire).

If one has very strong hunger pangs, experience dryness of

lips, throat and oral cavity, loses temper on missing meals and suffers from frequent episodes of acidity and heartburn, one may have *Tikshna agni* (overactive digestive fire).

If one has an inconsistent appetite, experiences bloating after meals, suffers from flatulence, abdominal pain and constipation, one may have *Vishama agni* (irregular digestive fire).

Acharya Charak mentions that when agni is *Sama* (functioning normally) the individual is happy and healthy. When it gets vitiated, the metabolism of the body gets disturbed, resulting in illness and disease. And when agni stops functioning, the individual dies. Therefore, agni is the *mool* (root) of human existence.

Signs of Healthy Agni	Signs of Weak Agni
• Timely cleansing of bowels and bladder • Good appetite • Good immunity and strength • Clear skin and lustre on the face • Normal functioning of all the sensory organs • Confident, affectionate, brave and logical personality	• Loss of appetite • Disturbed sleep • Lethargy and loss of enthusiasm • Depression and feeling of apathy • Constipation or diarrhoea • Fearful, confused, anxious and impatient personality

Science meets ancient wisdom

Modern medicine proves that there is constant division, multiplication and metabolism occurring in every cell of our body, from our birth till the time of our death. Agni provides the constant biological energy needed by the body to carry out these processes.

Ayurveda considers agni (digestive fire) to be of supreme importance in the process of *paka* (digestion) and metabolism. Food is essential for the maintenance of health, optimum digestion, absorption and assimilation of ingested food, according to Ayurveda. In the *Bramhasutras*, agni is considered to be a sign of life. Every parmanu or cell in our body is believed to be kindled with agni.

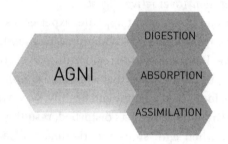

The role of agni

• Transforms food into energy, which performs all the crucial bodily functions
• Responsible for providing a healthy complexion, strength, nourishment, *ojas* (the essence of the tissues), *teja* (lustre) and prana (vital energy)

Depending upon the site of action and the function it performs, Acharya Charaka has mentioned 13 agnis: one Jatharagni, five Bhutagni and seven Dhatvagni.

Digestion: The ayurvedic perspective

The complete biological process of digestion, absorption and metabolism is governed by agni. It helps in the breakdown and release of energy from complex food material.

Jatharagni: This is the central digestive fire that oversees digestion in the entire gastrointestinal system. So, the seats of Jatharagni are the stomach and the duodenum of the small intestine. Ayurveda mentions the role of Jatharagni at three levels:

Kapha, pitta and vata evolve in our body as a result of these processes. Pitta corresponds to the digestive enzymes that work as catalysts in the digestion process. Jatharagni is the prime agni since it influences the functioning of the other 12 agnis.

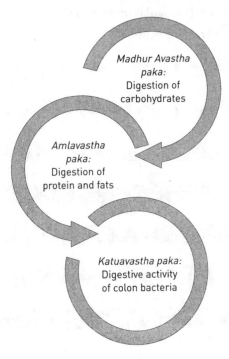

Bhutagni: From the small intestine, the digested materials reach the liver where they are converted into functional chemicals ready to be dispatched for use to various tissues. This is supervised by *Bhutagni*. Everything in our universe, including our body, is made of the five elements or *panchamahabutas*. There are five types of Bhutagnis, functioning in the five elements.

Parthiva in Earth	Apya in Water	Tejas in Fire	Vayavya in Air	Nabhasa in Space

According to Acharaya Charaka, every Bhutagni digests its respective element present in the ingested food.

Dhatvagni: This agni operates at the level of body tissues. According to acharyas, agni is present in the seven *dhatus* (tissues) of the body. They are known as:

Rasagni, which is present in the *rasa dhatu* (plasma)

Raktagni, which is present in the *rakta dhatu* (blood)

Mamsagni, which is present in the *mamsa dhatu* (muscles and skin)

Medagni, which is present in the *meda dhatu* (fat)

Asthyagni, which is present in the *asthi dhatu* (bones)

Majjagni, which is present in the *majja dhatu* (bone marrow)

Shukragni, which is present in the *shukra dhatu* (reproductive tissue)

These specialize in selecting and synthesizing portions from the food that are essential and nourishing to their tissue.

The end products of digestion are *Sara* and *Kitta*. While Sara is the essence that nourishes the doshas and dhatus (tissues), Kitta is the waste which must be thrown out of the body.

Ama: When your agni becomes weak, digestion becomes sub optimal. This results in the accumulation of toxins, which Ayurveda calls Ama. It causes sluggishness, poor appetite, nausea and constipation. Production of Ama is the root cause of all diseases.

Seven superfoods to strengthen agni

Dry ginger, black pepper, capsicum, mustard, turmeric, dates and raisins.

Seven yogic practices to improve digestion

Agnisara Kriya, Vajrasana, Bhujangasana, Halasana, Pavanamuktasana, Paschimottanasana and Dhanurasana.

UPAYOGASAMSTHA (DIETETIC RULES OF AYURVEDA)

For optimum digestion, *Charak Samhita* suggests the following rules. When adopted with a balanced diet, these factors help in strengthening agni and prevents the formation of ama.

Ushnam Bhunjit	Snigdham Bhunjit	Matravat Bhunjit	Jeerne Ashniyat	Veerya Aviruddha Ashniyat
• Consume food when it is warm, as it makes digestion easy and is more appetizing • Food, which is eaten hours after it is prepared takes longer to digest and is more likely to produce ama or toxins	• Food, which is unctuous and moist, is easily digested and nourishing. It facilitates vata to move downward, promotes growth, increases the acuity of senses and gives a healthy complexion • Dry foods may cause vatavyadhis (ailments caused due to vitiated vata) and (toxin) build-up	• Pay careful attention to the quantity of food. Always leave a quarter of your stomach empty, for vata-pitta-kapha to move. This avoids their imbalance • Overeating does not allow the tridoshas to move freely and leads to indigestion and production of Ama	• Ayurveda advises that the next meal must be taken only after the previous meal has been digested completely. This promotes longevity and keeps the doshas in balance • When this regime is not followed, the undigested food gets mixed with the partially digested food and causes an imbalance of doshas	• Foods that are incompatible with each other must be avoided. Only then will the digested materials optimally nourish the tissues • The consumption of contradictory foods is one of the major reasons behind skin diseases

A Dialogue With Your Body*

Every requirement of the body is conveyed to us via subtle bodily symptoms. Listening to our body is an active science, wherein by paying close attention to our bodily signals we can attain optimum health. Our bodies do not just exhibit symptoms, they also send signals through cravings, indicating a deficiency. For example, people who constantly crave sweets are generally deficient in the minerals magnesium and chromium, as well as the amino acid tryptophan. But one must know the difference between body signals and addictions! If you catch yourself craving unhealthy food, it means you need nutrients back in your diet. The best way to do this is to eat a well-balanced diet.

So, read your body! Try to observe the subtle changes that you sense are taking place within you:

Have you noticed a coating on your tongue?

A coating indicates poor digestion and accumulation of toxins in the body. The colour of the coating indicates the type of toxicity. Grey, black or brown, indicates the accumulation of vata toxins and imbalance. A yellow-, orange-, red-, or green-coloured layer indicate pitta toxins and imbalances. A whitish layer indicates kapha toxins and imbalances.

Bloated abdomen

Bloating can be caused by two factors: weak digestive fire or the formation of biotoxins i.e., ama. Ama can cause severe colic pain. Consumption of beans or fried foods, frozen or processed food, dairy products, fermented foods such as alcohol, incompatible food combinations such as milk and fruit or milk and fish can create gas in the intestine causing bloating and colic pain in the abdomen. This pain can also be exacerbated by improper food

---

Vibrant Ayurveda, Easy Ayurveda, Dr. Raghuram, Maharishi Ayurveda

habits such as eating your food in a hurry, lifestyle problems such as stress and sleep disturbances, not following a proper daily or seasonal regime, and the forcible suppression of natural urges like urination or defecation. A combination of cumin, coriander and fennel helps for better digestion. Turmeric, rock salt and asafoetida (hing) are excellent in eliminating gas and toxins.

Bad breath

Poor digestion, gum problems, dry mouth, cavities, poor oral hygiene, certain medications, respiratory issues, and foods such as onion, garlic and alcohol affect our breath. Turmeric, cumin, coriander, fennel, mint, asafoetida, black pepper, powdered ginger, cardamom, cinnamon, nutmeg and cayenne are some of the spices that aid digestion. They also help reduce ama from the body, which causes bad breath.

Low energy

Mental fatigue is associated with an imbalance in vata dosha. Emotional fatigue is caused by an imbalance in pitta dosha, while physical fatigue is caused by an imbalance in kapha dosha.

For mental fatigue, it is important to get ample and timely sleep, avoiding overwork and maintaining a vata reducing diet, besides practicing meditation.

To resolve emotional fatigue, try immersing oneself in hobbies hobbies and partake in good company along with enough rest.

For physical fatigue, eat light with some seasonings (such as turmeric, salt and long pepper) while doing moderate physical activity. It is important to sleep at 10 pm. The hours of sleep between 10 pm and 2 am will help replenish the body's vitality.

Tingling feet

Pain and tingling sensations in your feet indicate diabetic neuropathy and are due to the deterioration of vata dosha. The vitiation of pitta dosha causes a burning sensation. Drugs that pacify vata and pitta doshas are useful in the treatment of diabetic neuropathy. It is advised to include turmeric, cinnamon, warm water and ginkgo biloba in the diet. Exercise and a warm bath with massages of warm oil to increase circulation are prescribed.

MIND AND BODY CONNECT AS EXPRESSED IN THE CHARAK SAMHITA

Fever is known as a prolonged rise in body temperature usually around and above 98.6° F and is a symptom that the body is trying to fight an illness or infection. It is the body's feedback response in correspondence with the invasion of an unknown virus or bacteria in the body.

Fever as the first definite symptom of illness is also studied in the ancient texts and is expressed in the *Charak Samhita* as a phenomenon that occurs during birth and death, and also in conditions that are unhealthy and unhygienic. It can be natural or unnatural. Natural fever, as explained in the ancient texts, is easily curable in comparison and generally occurs in spring, due to aggravation of kapha, accumulated in winter and autumn or due to pitta vitiation, which is aggravated by hot and pungent foods. During such times, fasting can help cope up with these seasonal transitions.

Prayers, chanting hymns, devotion towards one's parents, respecting teachers, penance, truthfulness, observing rules, mantra repetitions, listening to the Vedas and the guru, were the traditional ways of coping with uneasiness and fever. These activities helped calm the mind and, in turn, reduced the fever since they are interconnected.

Fever as a reflection of the mind occurred when people are in low spirits. One can overcome it in various ways that can relief mental discomfort:

- **Fear, grief and passion:** Can be soothed by having conversations with loved ones, listening to calming words, spending time with loved ones and reducing vata vitiation.

- **Uncontrolled rage:** Can be pacified by alleviating pitta and listening to soothing words and indulging in favourite hobbies. Having your favourite food can also reduce this kind of fever.
- **Overthinking:** Can be pacified by distracting the individual with their favourite object or indulging in recreational activity.

According to Ayurveda, these feelings of unwholesomeness could also be alleviated by consuming Sattvik food.

1. **Gruels (Ragi, wheat, millets, rajgeera, coconut milk, palm sugar)**
   - Soupy warm food, cereals and good quality fats help pacify Vata. Here gruels fit in perfectly.
   - Gruels, coconut milk and palm sugar water help rehydrate the body when it loses an excess of water due to perspiration. The importance of hydration during fever is emphasized both in the ancient as well as modern times. Gruels are a great way to replenish nutrients and keep the body hydrated.

2. **Pulse soups (green gram, lentils, horse gram)**
   Pulses are a good source of protein. On sprouting, they are more easily digestible and are also rich in fiber. Consumption increases strength and immunity by lowering catabolism in the body.

3. **Gourds, especially ridge and bitter gourd**
   - Gourds are bitter, light and dry. They are known to be Kaphapittashāmaka, meaning they ease kapha and pitta aggravation.
   - Gourds kindle the agni in the stomach and increase the bile flow and aids digestion.
   - They are known to cleanse toxins in the body, aid digestion,

destroy kapha buildup, calm burning sensations and are anti-inflammatory.

- As is widely known, gourds have higher water content and can replenish water lost through sweating and polyuria (excessive urination) during fever.

3

RITUCHARYA

Tasya Shitadiya Ahaarbalam Varnascha Vardhate.
Tasyartusatmayam Vaditam Chestaharvyapasrayam

The strength and complexion of an individual who knows the suitable diet and regimen for every season and practices it accordingly is enhanced.

—Charak Samhita, Tripathi B.

Ritu means 'season' and Charya means 'lifestyle' or 'regime'. Ayurveda states that just as the change of seasons affects our external environment (the leaves, flowers, winds and soil), they also affect our internal environment—our body and mind. So, a change in dietary and lifestyle practices according to seasons becomes essential to maintain the body homeostasis. It also prepares the body to fight seasonal infections and ailments.

CLASSIFICATION OF SEASONS (AS PER INDIAN TOPOGRAPHY)

According to Ayurveda, the year is divided into two, based on the direction in which the sun moves. The period during which the sun moves through the northern solstice is called Uttarayana. When the sun moves through the southern solstice it is called Dakshinayana. Each solstice comprises three ritus or seasons.

DIETARY AND LIFESTYLE GUIDELINES ACCORDING TO SEASONS

Uttarayana (Adana Kala)	Dakshinayana (Visarga Kala)
Shishir (winter), Vasanta (spring) and Grishma (summer)	Varsha (monsoon), Sarata (autumn) and Hemanta (late autumn)
• Sun and wind are strong • Predominant properties: Tikta (bitter), Kashaya (astringent), Rasa (taste) • The body tends to become dry and strength is reduced	• The Earth cools down, winds turn cool • Predominant properties: Amla (sour), Lavana (salty) and Madhura (sweet) • Body strength is enhanced

DIETARY AND LIFESTYLE GUIDELINES ACCORDING TO SEASONS

Shishir (Winter)	
• Kapha accumulates, • Agni is strong	**Diet:** Prefer sour foods such as Indian gooseberry or amla. Cereals, pulses, gram flour, rice, corn, ginger, garlic, sugarcane, milk and milk products. Avoid bitter and astringent tasting foods.
	Lifestyle: Oil/powder/paste massages, bathing with lukewarm water, sunbathing and wearing warm clothes is recommended.
Vasanta (Spring) • Kapha dosha gets vitiated • Agni is of medium strength	**Diet:** Consume easily digestible foods such as cereals, old barley, wheat, rice, lentils and green gram. Bitter, pungent and astringent foods are beneficial. Honey should be included.
	Lifestyle: Bathing with lukewarm water and exercising is beneficial. Avoid sleeping during the day.
Grishma (Summer) • Vata dosha gets deposited • Agni is mild	**Diet:** Consume easily digestible foods that is sweet, unctuous and cold. Rice, lentils, buttermilk, fruit juices, soups, along with plenty of water is advised. Avoid pungent, sour and warm foods.
	Lifestyle: Stay indoors during this season in a cool environment. Apply sandlewood or Fuller's earth on the body to keep it cool. Wear light-coloured clothes. Short naps can be taken during the day. One can also try moonbathing. Avoid vigorous exercises during this period.

Varsha (monsoon)	Diet: Prefer sour, salty and unctuous foods such as old barely, rice, wheat and soups. Boiled water should be consumed. Avoid excessive liquids and food that is difficult to digest, such as meat.
• Vata dosha gets vitiated • Agni gets affected	
	Lifestyle: Have bath with lukewarm water. Rub your body with oil after bath. Avoid getting wet in the rain. Avoid exertion.
Sharat (Autumn) • Pitta dosha gets vitiated • Agni becomes active	Diet: Prefer sweet, bitter and easily digestible foods having cooling properties. Wheat, green gram, honey and gourds are recommended. Avoid hot, bitter, sweet and astringent foods which are fatty. Avoid curd.
	Lifestyle: Eat only when hungry. Rub the chandan paste on your body. Moonbathing is recommneded. Avoid long exposure to sunlight. It is advised to avoid sleeping during the day and overeating.
Hemant (Late autumn) • Pitta dosha gets pacified • Agni is active	Diet: Consume unctuous, sweet, sour and salty foods. Rice, flour preparations, green gram, milk and milk products, sugarcane products, fermented products and sesame must be included in the diet. Avoid cold, dry and light foods. Cold drinks are prohibited.
	Lifestyle: Exercise, massage the head and body, wear warm clothing and stay in warm places. Avoid going out when there are strong winds. It is advised to avoid sleeping during the day.

DINCHARYA: THE DISCIPLINED DAILY ROUTINE

'No matter how awesome it may be from a materialistic perspective, it will not lead us to prosperity and well-being unless we also drive the same with the right values and processes that sustain our collective harmony and prosperity.'

Keeping the baton of preventive lifestyle high, Ayurveda lists a few effective strategies: Dincharya (daily regimen), Ritucharya (seasonal regimen), Sadvitta (good moral conduct), and Ashtanga yoga (eightfold path to salvation). These practices form crucial pillars to maintain a healthy body and mind.

Dincharya is the Sanskrit word for a daily regimen. In Ayurveda, kala (time) is considered to be the cause of disease. The passage of time fosters diseases. Therefore, Ayurvedic acharyas have suggested lifestyle changes in daily routine along with ahara (dietary) and vihara (behaviour) modifications to live a balanced and healthy life.

VARIOUS DINCHARYA MODALITIES AND THEIR BENEFICIAL EFFECTS ON BODY AND MIND

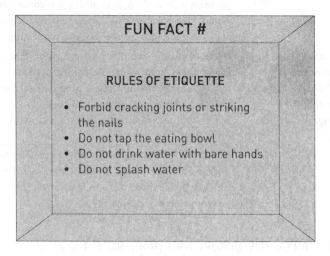

FUN FACT

RULES OF ETIQUETTE

- Forbid cracking joints or striking the nails
- Do not tap the eating bowl
- Do not drink water with bare hands
- Do not splash water

Here is how an ideal daily routine should be, according to the teachings of Ayurveda.

Brahmamuhurta-jagarana: Wake up just before sunrise	Wake up 90 minutes before sunrise to experience fresh atmosphere that is full of oxygen. This is the perfect time to practise yoga and meditation. It releases serotonin, which makes us feel positive and happy.

Ushapan (drinking warm water)	Consume 1-2 glasses of lukewarm water on waking up to clear the intestines and facilitate purgation.
Darpanenamukhasayavalokana: Look at yourself in the mirror	Look in a mirror to check for any signs of inflammation or abnormality.
Malotsarga (defecation and urination)	Attend to nature's call in the morning. This improves digestion and keeps the skin healthy.
Achamana (wash hands)	Washing hands after excretion, eating, crying, sneezing and travelling is essential for personal hygiene and for prevention of infections.
Danta dhavana (teeth brushing)	Chewing on neem tree twigs releases margosine, which acts like an antibacterial. Brush your teeth twice a day in vertical direction. This is an essential oral hygiene practice.
Jihva nirlekhana (tongue cleaning)	Scraping the tongue with a copper, silver or iron tongue scraper stimulates appetite and removes bad breath. It removes the toxic layer on the tongue.
Snehagandusha dharana (Oil pulling)	Oil pulling keeps the oral cavity healthy and strengthens the muscles of the jaw and cheeks.
Dhumpana (inhaling medicated fumes)	When medicated herbs are lit, they produce fumes. Inhaling them stimulates the respiratory tract and clears the nasal passages.
Mukha netraprakshalana (washing your face and eyes)	Washing your eyes and face freshens you up. It also prevents eye infections.
Sugandhitadravyadharana Tambulasevana (Use mouth freshener and betel leaves)	This activates the taste buds and regulates salivation.
Anjana (application of collyrium)	This keeps the eyes healthy and makes them shine. It prevents itching, burning and watering of eyes.

Nasya (oily nasal drops)	This practice increases the strength of the sense organs, gives good sleep and improves the breathing process.
Vyayama (physical exercise)	Regular practise of yoga, meditation and pranayama is advised. Exercise improves blood circulation and supplies oxygen to different parts of the body.
Abhyanga (body massage with oil)	Oil massage improves blood circulation throughout the body. Additionally, performing accupressure releases endorphins.
Snana (Bathing)	Bathing improves appetite, mood, motivation and removes sweat, dead skin and other impurities on the surface of the body.
Anulepana (inhaling aromas)	Inhaling soothing and pleasing aroma, using incense, cheers up the mind and vitalizes the senses.
Sandhyopasana (Worshipping the divine)	Remembering the supreme energy and praying grounds us, preparing us for the day ahead.

INTELLIGENT SNACKING

A) BREAKFAST/EXERCISE MEALS

1. PORRIDGE

AMARANTH AND MUNG PORRIDGE

Aromatic mung pudding is enriched with the umami freshness from amaranth, leaves and spices.

Skill level	Moderate
Serving size	2
Place of origin	India
Season most suited for consumption	All seasons
Rich in nutrients	Calcium, phosphorus, zinc, copper

Know your nutrition

Green gram (Mung): It is a plant-based source of protein, ideal for vegetarians and vegans. It is a source of zinc, folate and copper. Sprouting the gram increases the amount of Vitamin C by three times, this helps in defending against several chronic, age-related diseases. It is helpful in weight loss as it is low in fat and has dietary fiber.

Green peas: These are one of the best plant-based sources of protein, which is a major reason why they are so filling. Along with a high amount of fiber they reduce appetite and promote feelings of satiation. They contain a decent amount of heart-healthy minerals, such as magnesium, potassium and calcium, and even help to regulate the blood sugar levels.

Favourable for conditions

Bone health, Weight loss, Irritable bowel syndrome and Gluten-free diets

Calorie count

Serving size	Energy (Kcal)	Carbohydrate (gm)	Protein (gm)	Fats (gm)	Calcium (mg)	Phosphorus (mg)
1	186	20.6	6.6	6.3	132.4	106.4
2	373	41.2	13.2	12.6	264.9	212.8

Serving size	Total fiber (mg)	Ómega-30 (mg)	Zinc (mg)	Copper (mg)	
1	6.3	99.8	0.7	0.4	
2	12.5	199.6	1.4	0.8	

Ingredients

Whole amaranth	30 gm
Sprouted mung	30 gm
Green peas	25 gm
Carrot	25 gm
Oil	1 tsp
Ginger paste	2 tsp
Mustard seed	1 tsp
Cumin seed	2 tsp
Sesame (til) seed	15 gm
Curry leaves	3-4
Turmeric powder	1 tsp
Coriander powder	1 tsp
Salt	¼ tsp

Method

- Boil the entire amaranth. In a pan add oil, mustard seeds, cumin seeds, curry leaves, til seeds and ginger paste. After 10–20 seconds, add corn, green peas and carrot. Sauté for 3–4 minutes.
- Add sprouted mung and sauté for another 4–5 minutes. Add amaranth, salt, turmeric powder and coriander powder. Mix well for another 4–5 minutes. Serve in a bowl and add coriander.

Healthy cooking tips

- After boiling the amaranth, do not throw away the water. It can be used for other purposes including kneading the dough.

- Amaranth is a good source of calcium and can also be used to make chikki and ladoo.
- Spouted mung can also be replaced by matki.

❦

DELICIOUS PORRIDGE

Ancient Indian porridge makes for a wholesome meal with wholesome ingredients like barley, apples, dates and nuts.

Skill level	Easy
Serving size	3
Place of origin	Indian
Season most suited for consumption	All seasons
Rich in nutrients	Fiber, magnesium, iron, potassium, vitamin C, calcium

Know your nutrition

- **Barley:** It has beta-glucan, a soluble fiber that may help lower cholesterol and improve blood sugar control. It contains antioxidants such as vitamin E, beta-carotene, lutein and zeaxanthin, which help protect against and repair cell damage caused by oxidative stress. It has shown to improve symptoms of ulcerative colitis (an inflammatory bowel disease), relieve constipation and increase probiotic activity. It is an excellent diuretic and can be used as a detox and for urinary tract infections and renal issues.
- **Chikoo:** It is an energy dense fruit and a good source of vitamins C and A. It also contains minerals like magnesium, potassium, phosphorous and iron. The fruit helps maintain bone mineral density, relieves constipation, fights inflammation, controls blood pressure and prevents cancers of the oral cavity.

- **Cow's milk:** It is an ideal source of protein for vegetarians, which gets easily absorbed in the body. It is rich in calcium and vitamin D, which strengthen our bones. The presence of vitamin B12 makes it important for brain health. It is also good for your heart.

Favourable for conditions

Pregnancy, Bone health, Hypertension, Cardiac health, Immunity and Stress.

Calorie count

Serving size	Energy (Kcal)	Carbohydrate (gm)	Protein (gm)	Fats (gm)	Calcium (mg)	Phosphorus (mg)
1	232	32	6.8	8.2	147.1	104.3
3	698	96	20.3	24.6	441.2	312.9
Serving size	Iron (mg)	Potassium (mg)	Magnesium (mg)	Total Fiber (mg)	Omega-3 (mg)	Vitamin C (mg)
1	0.4	249.9	13.5	5.7	49.5	5.9
3	1.3	749.7	40.5	17.1	148.4	17.6

Ingredients

Barley	¼ cup
Cow's milk	2 cup
Dates (soaked)	3
Almonds	7-8
Apple	½ cup
Chikoo	½ cup

Method

- Heat milk in a vessel. Bring it to the boil, then add barley, chopped almonds, dates, apple and chikoo.
- Let the mixture boil till the barley is cooked. Then take it off the heat and serve it in a bowl.

Healthy cooking tips

- Do not overcook the barley.
- Cow's milk also contains a high amount of saturated fat and cholesterol, which can increase the risk of heart diseases. So, you can replace cow milk with goat milk or soya milk.
- Dates can be added as a natural sweetener to many desserts.
- Apple should be consumed with the skin.

❧

ODANA (RICE PUDDING)

A delightful Ayurvedic barley pudding recipe that harks back to prehistoric India. Odana is highly nutritive and aids in digestion.

Skill level	Easy
Serving size	1
Place of origin	India
Season most suited for consumption	All seasons
Rich in nutrients	Protein, Calcium

Know your nutrition

Nutmeg (Jaifhal): It helps to stop diarrhoea (in low dose), detoxify the body and stimulate the brain. It has antioxidant, antimicrobial and antifungal properties. However, consuming too much of nutmeg results in sudden attack, irregular heart palpitations and vomiting.

Cardamom (Elaichi): It can be used to treat respiratory and gastrointestinal (GI) tract infections along with kidney and urinary disorders (increases the frequency of urination). It reduces all kinds of inflammations, even of eyelids and antibacterial infections of teeth and gums. It is an antidote for both snake and scorpion venom and also used for food poisoning. It is also used as a mouth freshener.

Favourable for conditions

Bone disorders, Heart disease, Brain disease

Calorie count

Serving Size	Energy (Kcal)	Carbohydrate (gm)	Protein (gm)	Fats (gm)	Calcium (mg)	Phosphorus (mg)
1	290	40.1	9.0	9.1	200.6	146.5

Serving Size	Total Fiber (mg)	Omega-3 (mg)
1	3	48

Ingredients

Rice	30 gm
Milk	200 ml
Raisins	1 tsp
Cardamom	2 no
Honey	1 tsp
Nutmeg powder	1 tsp

Method

- Rinse rice in cold water. In a pan, add barley and 1 cup of water. Cover it with a lid.
- Bring the mix to a boil.
- Then drain the rice and add it to the pan.
- Add milk, honey, cardamom and raisins.
- Bring the mix to a simmer, cover and cook until the rice is tender and the milk has thickened, stirring occasionally.
- Garnish with nutmeg powder.

Healthy cooking tips

- Can use almond milk or coconut milk as an alternative.
- Can use barley as an alternative to rice.
- Skim the cream and then use the milk for drinking.

- Cow's milk also contains a high amount of saturated fat and cholesterol, which can increase the risk of heart diseases. You can replace cow's milk with goat milk or soya milk.

☙

RAGI SATVA/PUDDING

A wholesome Konkani style pudding, it is easy to make and abundant in healthy ingredients.

Skill level	Easy
Serving size	6
Place of origin	Goa, India
Season most suited for consumption	All seasons
Rich in nutrients	Iron, vitamins, omega-3 fatty acid, magnesium

Know your nutrition

Coconut is low in carbohydrates and high in fiber, which helps stabilize blood sugar. It also has an anti-diabetic effect due to its arginine content. High in antioxidants, it prevents oxidative damage. It also has a beneficial effect on heart health and is good for skin and hair health.

Favourable for conditions

Bone health, Pregnancy, Children, Senior citizens, Skin and hair health.

Calorie count

Serving Size	Energy (Kcal)	Carbohydrate (gm)	Protein (gm)	Fats (gm)	Calcium (mg)
1	255	41.8	2.6	7.9	80.3
6	1533	250.9	15.5	47.5	482.2

Serving Size	Phosphorus (mg)	Total Fiber (mg)	Omega-3 (mg)	Potassium (mg)	Magnesium (mg)
1	50.9	2.7	8.2	245.6	31.1
6	305.8	16.7	49.5	1473.8	186.6

Ingredients

Ragi flour	1 cup
Grated coconut	1 cup
Jaggery	1 cup
Raisins	1 tbsp
Cashew nuts, broken into pieces	2 tbsp
Cardamom powder	½ tsp
Salt	½ tsp
Ghee	1 tsp

Method

- Soak the ragi for 5–6 hours.
- Now, grind the coconut with a little water into a smooth, even paste. Extract coconut milk using muslin cloth or a strainer.
- Soak the jaggery in the coconut milk, and set aside.
- Grind the ragi with sufficient water to get a smooth paste.
- Put the ground ragi paste in a muslin cloth or any other strainer and extract the juice. Strain the juice again.
- Keep the ragi juice aside for ½ hour. All the excess water will accumulate at the top.
- Add the ragi juice, coconut milk and jaggery in a thick-bottomed pan and cook over a low flame, stirring continuously.
- As it starts thickening, add raisins, cashew nuts, cardamom powder and salt. Then mix well.
- Once it has thickened, transfer it to a flat-bottomed plate greased with ghee.
- Let it cool. It will further thicken and achieve pudding consistency

- Cut the ragi satva into squares and serve.

Healthy cooking tips

- Jowar /bajra flour can be used instead of ragi.
- In the summer season, you can also use mango as an alternative to ragi and make mango pudding.

2. PANCAKE/CHILA

MUNCHY GREEN PROTEIN MUNG DAL CHILA

A nourishing version of savoury pancake with fresh green leaves and protein-rich Sattvik mung dal.

Skill level	Easy
Serving size	4
Place of origin	India
Season most suited for consumption	All seasons
Rich in nutrients	Potassium, Fiber, Calcium, Iron, Magnesium, Phosphorus, Vitamin C

Know your nutrition

- **Green gram (Mung):** It is a plant-based source of protein, ideal for vegetarians and vegans. It is also a source of zinc, folate and copper. Sprouting the gram increases the amount of Vitamin C by three times. This helps in defending against several chronic, age-related diseases. It is helpful in weight loss as it is low in fat and has dietary fiber.
- **Coriander (Dhania):** It reduces cholesterol deposition by lowering cholesterol levels and blood sugar. It is good for digestion as it contains high insoluble fiber and reduces urinary tract infection. It is rich in vitamin C vitamin K and

antioxidants. It also has the ability to ease muscles spasms and flatulence.

- **Groundnut oil (Singdana/Mungfali ka Tel):** It has vitamin E that protects from oxidative damage and reduces the risk of heart disease, cholesterol and maintains skin health. It is rich in omega-9 and omega-6 fatty acids and polyphenols like resveratrol that helps to maintain blood pressure, improves immune health, lowers Alzheimer's disease and prevents cancer.

Favourable for conditions

Weight loss, Anemia, Diabetes, Hypertension, Cardiac Health, Constipation

Calorie count

Serving Size	Energy (Kcal)	Carbohydrate (gm)	Protein (gm)	Fats (gm)	Calcium (mg)	Phosphorus (mg)
1	250	35.6	13	1	24.8	4.8
4	1001	142.4	52.2	4.2	99.3	19.3
Serving Size	Iron (mg)	Sodium (mg)	Potassium (mg)	Magnesium (mg)	Total Fiber (mg)	Omega-3 (mg)
1	1.2	437.5	428.7	22.1	7.1	23.2
4	4.8	1749.9	1715	88.3	28.3	93.2

Ingredients

Mung dal, soaked for 3 hours	250 gm
Coriander leaves	Few
Ginger	1 inch
Groundnut oil	1 tbsp
Salt	½ tsp

Method

- Grind soaked mung dal into a smooth paste.
- Add coriander and ginger and grind one more time in the blender to get a bright green colour and a smooth paste.

- Mix well and make it as a dosa batter consistency.
- Coat the tawa with a layer of oil.
- Take a small portion of the batter and pour it on the hot tawa and let it cook one side.
- Gently flip when one side has browned it with chutney of your choice.

Healthy cooking tips

- Wash mung dal well and discard the water. Discarding water may reduce bloating and can also reduce uric acid levels.
- Do not sieve besan for the recipe.
- Groundnut oil is a good source of monounsaturated fat (MUFA), so it is a healthier cooking oil.

MUNG DAL CORIANDER PANCAKE

A vibrant and appetizing all-time recipe.

Skill level	Moderate
Serving size	4
Place of origin	India
Season most suited for consumption	All seasons
Rich in nutrients	Protein, Dietary fiber, B-complex vitamins, vitamin C, sodium, potassium, magnesium, phosphorus, selenium, antioxidants

Know your nutrition

Mung gram (Yellow mung dal): It is a plant-based source of protein, ideal for vegetarians and vegans. It is a good source of zinc and vitamin B1. It is light and very easy to digest. It helps in stabilizing blood sugar.

Brown rice: Brown rice is a whole grain and a good source of magnesium, phosphorus, selenium, thiamine, niacin, vitamin B6, and manganese, and the fiber in it helps manage cholesterol, moves waste through the digestive tract, gives satiety and helps to prevent the formation of blood clots.

Coriander (Dhania): It reduces cholesterol deposition by lowering cholesterol levels and blood sugar. It is good for digestion as it contains high insoluble fiber and reduces urinary tract infection. It is rich in vitamin C, hence possess antioxidant activity and vitamin K. It has the ability to remove muscle spasm, as rich in antioxidants and flatulence.

Favourable for conditions

Weight loss, Diabetes, Children, Adolescents, Gluten intolerance, Senior citizens, Pregnant and lactating women

Calorie count

Serving Size	Energy (Kcal)	Carbohydrate (gm)	Total Fiber (mg)	Protein (gm)	Fats (gm)	Omega-3 (mg)
1	247	37.1	6.2	10.9	2.7	20.4
4	988	148.4	24.7	43.4	10.7	81.4
Serving Size	Calcium (mg)	Phosphorus (mg)	Sodium (mg)	Potassium (mg)	Iron (mg)	Vitamin C (mg)
1	20.4	98.5	424.2	351.2	1	0.2
4	81.8	394	1696.7	1404.7	4.2	0.8

Ingredients

Brown rice	¼ cup
Mung dal	2 cup
Coriander	¼ cup
Filtered rice bran oil	½ tbsp

Grated coconut	¼ cup
Pink salt	1 tsp
Water	½ cup

Method

- Soak the brown rice and mung dal for about 3 hours.
- Add the soaked brown rice, mung dal, coriander leaves and little water in the bowl of a food processor and whizz to form a thick batter. Season as per taste.
- Add freshly grated coconut.
- Heat a tawa and layer it with rice bran oil. Pour one cup of the batter on the tawa and spread it a bit.
- As soon as bubbles start to appear on the upper side, flip it and cook the other side until the pancake turns brown.
- Garnish it with coriander, coconut flakes and serve it with fresh mint chutney.

Healthy cooking tips

- Good alternative to brown rice is black rice.
- Do not strain the rice water. Use it in other preparations like soups.
- Soaked mung dal for at least 4–5 hours. Wash well and then boil it. Sprouting mung is a nutritive alternative. Wash the coriander leaves before using. It is a versatile herb used for making chutney, garnishing dishes. It can remove spasm of smooth muscles as it is rich in antioxidants and reduces flatulence.
- Avoid using excess oil for pan frying.

OATS AND SPROUT PANCAKE

Wholesome nourishing oats pancakes are perfect for snacks with the goodness of sprouts.

Skill level	Moderate
Serving size	2
Place of origin	India
Season most suited for consumption	All seasons
Rich in nutrients	Protein, Calcium, Fiber, Zinc, Copper

Know your nutrition

Sprouts are alkaline; hence they should be consumed to balance the pH. Sprouts are good for diabetic patients, and helps increase the protein content. Sprouts also have a high level of vitamin C.

Favourable for conditions

Diabetes, Bone health, Children, Weight loss

Calorie count

Serving Size	Energy (Kcal)	Carbohydrate (gm)	Protein (gm)	Fats (gm)	Omega-3 (mg)
1	218	23.7	7.4	7.5	28.5
2	436	47.4	14.8	15.0	57
Serving Size	Calcium (mg)	Phosphorus (mg)	Total Fiber (mg)	Zinc (mg)	Copper (mg)
1	142.8	102.0	5.7	0.6	0.3
2	285.6	204.0	11.4	1.2	0.6

Ingredients

Oats flour	30 gm
Gram flour	15 gm
Sprouts	30 gm
Capsicum	25 gm
Carrot	25 gm
Salt	1/4 tsp
Cumin seed	2 tsp

Coriander powder	1 tsp
Black til seed	15 gm
Oil	2 tsp

Method

- Grind the sprout into a paste.
- In a bowl add oats flour, gram flour, and little water. Mix it well.
- Add the sprout paste along with all other ingredients. Mix it well. Make a paste of pouring consistency.
- Take a ladleful of paste and pour it on a pan. Let it cook for 1-2 minutes and flip it.
- Cook until it becomes golden brown and then serve it.

Healthy cooking tips

- Matki sprout can be used instead of mung sprout.
- Til seeds can also be sprouted as sprouting improves its nutritional content.
- Use steel-cut rolled oats and not processed oats or instant oats.
- Oats if used as a powder in a soup or vegetable should be nicely dry roasted before powdering, which can then be added to the preparation as a thickening agent. E.g.: In dals and soups.

❧

SAGO CHILA

Delicious and nutritional sago chila that satisfy the cravings.

Skill level	Easy
Serving size	5
Place of origin	India
Season most suited for consumption	All seasons
Rich in nutrients	Fiber, Folate, Potassium, Calcium, Magnesium, Iron, Phosphorus

Know your nutrition

Sago: It is rich in energy, gluten-free and non-allergic. It is a good source of dietary fibers that helps prevent digestion issues, relieves gas, bloating, constipation and also rebalance the healthy gut bacteria. It contains potassium that helps to control blood pressure. It is rich in vitamin B6 and folate. It is a great source of protein that helps repair damaged cells and tissues and helps in the growth of the cells. It is high in calcium, magnesium, calcium and iron, which help to make bones strong and improve their density and lower the risk of arthritis and osteoporosis.

Samo rice: It has high nutritional value and gluten-free. It is easily digestible and provides satiety. It has high fiber content. It is less in calories, so helps to lose weight. It can be consumed by diabetic patients as it has less sugar. It is high in protein, which helps in growth and maintenance of cells.

Sunflower oil (Surajmukhi ka tel): It contains vitamin E that protects cells from age-related damage and strengthens your immune system. It has anti-inflammatory properties that reduce the risk of rheumatoid arthritis and asthma. It also helps to reduce high cholesterol levels and heart disease.

Favourable for conditions

Children, Athletes, Fasting Food

Calorie count

Serving Size	Carbohydrate (gm)	Protein (gm)	Fats (gm)	Calcium (mg)	Phosphorus (mg)
1	65.9	3	0.5	12.3	64.8
5	329.4	15.1	2.6	61.4	324.1
Serving Size	Iron (mg)	Potassium (mg)	Magnesium (mg)	Total Fiber (mg)	Omega-3 (mg)
1	0.4	86.4	18.6	1.2	4.3
5	2.1	433.2	93	6	21.7

Ingredients

Sago	1 cup
Samo rice	1 cup
Coriander leaves	1 tbsp
Cumin seeds	2 tsp
Sunflower oil	1 tsp

Method

- Soak sago in water for about 3 hours and soak samo rice the overnight. Blend sago and samo rice separately. Pour both the puree in a bowl, add coriander leaves, cumin seeds and water and mix to a thin, watery consistency.
- Smear a pan with oil. Take a ladleful of the batter and pour it on the pan. Let it cook for 2-3 minutes, or until....slightly brown and serve it with any chutney of choice.

Healthy cooking tips

- Sago and samo rice can be soaked in warm water.
- Sunflower oil is non-volatile oil, has a very high smoke point used mostly for cooking and frying.
- Coriander is a versatile herb used in making chutney, garnishing dishes. It can remove spasm of the smooth muscles as it is rich in antioxidants and reduces flatulence.

❧

SARAMYA

Saramya (rice pancake) is a scrumptious savoury pancake

Skill level	Moderate
Serving size	1
Place of origin	Gujarat, India
Season most suited for consumption	Spring, Summer

Rich in nutrients

White rice is a good source of magnesium, phosphorus, manganese, selenium, iron, folic acid, thiamine and niacin. Besan is rich in protein, iron, folate, copper and antioxidants.

Know your nutrition

White rice is a good source of magnesium, phosphorus, manganese, selenium, iron, folic acid, thiamine and niacin and additionally, its low fiber content may help with digestive issues.

Favourable for conditions

Digestion, Diabetic patients

Calorie count

Serving Size	Energy (Kcal)	Carbohydrate (gm)	Total Fiber (mg)	Protein (gm)	Fats (gm)	Omega-3 (mg)
1	144	26.92	1.02	2.62	1.83	5.92
Serving Size	Calcium (mg)	Phosphorous (mg)	Selenium (mg)	Magnesium (mg)	Manganese (mg)	Folic acid (mcg)
1	4.68	24.66	0.775	6.725	0.39	1.325

Ingredients

Rice cooked	2 cups
Turmeric	1 tsp
Salt	¼ tsp
Besan flour	1 tbsp
Filtered oil	1 tbsp

Method

- Put the cooked rice in the bowl, add all the spices and besan flour and mix it well.

- Then divide the mixture into 5-6 portions and roll it.
- Flatten each portion and make it like a mini pancake
- Heat the tawa and then smear some oil on it.
- Put the mini pancake on the tawa and roll it up and down till both sides become slightly brown.
- Repeat the steps for all the other portions and serve hot with chutneys or dip.

Healthy cooking tips

- Rice has low fiber content that can help with digestive issues.
- Use parboiled rice instead of basmati rice.
- Alternatively, brown rice or black rice can be used.
- Do not strain the rice water away. Use it in other preparations like soups.
- Besan is a plant-based source of protein, ideal for vegetarians and vegans. It is a source of iron, folate and copper and provides satiety and energy. It stabilizes blood sugar, which prevents diabetes. It also contains phytochemicals called saponins that act as antioxidants.

VEGETABLE HANDVO

Delicious savoury cake with the incorporation of fresh vegetables such as carrot, spinach and bottle gourd.

Skill level	Moderate
Serving size	2
Place of origin	Gujarat, India
Season most suited for consumption	All seasons
Rich in nutrients	Protein, Phosphorus, Fiber, Beta carotene

Know your nutrition

Mung gram (yellow mung dal): It is a plant-based source of protein, ideal for vegetarians and vegans. It is a good source of zinc and vitamin B1. It is light and very easy to digest. It helps in stabilizing blood sugar.

Bottle gourd (Lauki): Bottle gourd is a modest source of vitamin C, which is one of the most powerful antioxidants. It helps the body to fight against free radicals, cancer, and inflammation. It is even a good source of calcium and has a high content of water. It is rich in dietary fiber that helps in curing indigestion and constipation.

Favourable for conditions

Diabetes, Pregnancy, Lactation

Calorie count

Serving Size	Energy (Kcal)	Carbohydrate (gm)	Protein (gm)	Fats (gm)	Calcium (mg)
1	196	18.7	7.3	8.03	101.2
2	393	37.4	14.6	16.1	202.4
Serving Size	Phosphorus (mg)	Total Fiber (mg)	Omega-3 (mg)	Beta carotene (mcg)	Vitamin C (mg)
1	99.2	8.7	189.4	897.9	2.9
2	198.4	17.4	378.8	1795.8	5.8

Ingredients

Mungdal	60 gm
Carrot	25 gm
Peas	25 gm
Spinach	50 gm
Bottle gourd	50 gm
Oil	2 tsp

Mustard seed	2 tsp
Cumin seed	2 tsp
Curry leaves	4–5
Salt	¼ tsp
Til seed	7 gm
Bay leaf	2

Method

- Soak the dal overnight and grind it in a paste. Add salt and all the vegetables and mix well.
- In a pan add oil, cumin seed, and mustard seed, til seed, curry leaves, bay leaf, and 2 ladleful of batter.
- Cover and let it cook for 3-4 minutes, then flip it and cook until it becomes golden brown.
- Serve hot.

Healthy cooking tips

- Other vegetables like fenugreek, capsicum and corn can also be added.
- Handvo can also be made from tur dal or green mung dal.
- Sprouted til seeds can also be added as sprouting improves its nutritional content.

WATERMELON RIND PANCAKE

An enjoyable easy to make a naturally sweetened pancake with zero-waste impact.

Skill level	Easy
Serving size	1
Place of origin	South India, India
Season most suited for consumption	Spring, Summer

Rich in nutrients   Potassium, Magnesium, and
                           Antioxidants

Know your nutrition

Watermelon rind: It is a rich source of fiber, helps maintain regular bowel movements and may help reduce the risk of developing diseases of the colon.

Jaggery: Jaggery is loaded with antioxidants and minerals like zinc and selenium, which help prevent free-radicals (responsible for early aging). Due to richness in essential nutrients, it is effective in solving menstrual problems. Jaggery is rich in iron and folate, which help in preventing anemia. It also boosts intestinal strength due to its high magnesium content.

Favourable for conditions

Irritable Bowel Syndrome, Children, Adolescents

Calorie count

Serving Size	Energy (Kcal)	Carbohydrate (gm)	Total Fiber (mg)	Protein (gm)	Fats (gm)	Omega-3 (mg)
1	287	34.3	1.9	3.7	16.5	9.3
Serving Size	Calcium (mg)	Potassium (mg)	Sodium (mg)	Magnesium (mg)	Phosphorous (mcg)	Folate (mg)
1	11.7	212	1752	5.5	30.3	1.8

Ingredients

Chopped watermelon rind	2½ cups
Parboiled rice	1 cup
Coconut milk	½ cup
Jaggery	2 gm
Himalayan pink salt (Saindhav namak)	1 gram

Method

- Add all the ingredients in a blender and process to a smooth but slightly grainy paste.
- Add water to make thin and runny.
- Grease the pan and pour a ladleful of the batter. Let it cook for 2-3 minutes.
- Flip the pancake and let it cook for 1-2 minutes. Serve shot.

Healthy cooking tips

- Use parboiled rice instead of basmati rice.
- Alternatively, brown rice or black rice can be used.

B. SNACKS

1. CHAAT

DAHI TIKKI CHAT

Scrumptious Indian chat delicacy that has a combination of sweet and tangy flavours.

Skill level	Moderate
Serving size	2
Place of origin	India
Season most suited for consumption	All seasons
Rich in nutrients	Calcium, Iron, Fiber, Beta carotene

Know your nutrition

Curd: Curd is rich in lactococcus lactis, which encourages the growth of healthy gut flora and promotes digestion. It improves skeletal muscle as it is rich in calcium content. It is a good probiotic food that keeps ecosystem balance and prevents the activity of harmful micro-organisms. The bioactive protein in curd reduces blood pressure and cholesterol levels.

Pomegranate (Anaar): Pomegranates contain punicalagins and punicic acid that are responsible for most of their health benefits. Pomegranate seeds prevent forming clots and coagulating. Pomegranates are packed with nutrients such as vitamin A, C, fiber, copper. It helps boosts immunity and has anti-bacterial and anti-inflammatory properties and reduces urinary tract infections. It also relieves constipation and reduces dental caries.

Favourable for conditions

Bone health, Children, Pregnancy, Adolescent

Calorie count

Serving Size	Energy (Kcal)	Carbohydrate (gm)	Protein (gm)	Fats (gm)	Calcium (mg)
1	235	39.6	4	5.9	131.5
2	469	79.2	8	11.8	263
Serving Size	Phosphorus (mg)	Total Fiber (mg)	Omega-3 (mg)	Iron (mg)	Beta carotene (mcg)
1	67	6.9	72.2	3	3026.6
2	134	13.8	144.4	6	6053.2

Ingredients

Sweet potato	100 gm
Peas	25 gm
Oil	2 tsp
Cumin seed	1 tsp
Salt	¼ tsp
Turmeric powder	1 tsp
Coriander powder	1 tsp
Curd	100 gm

Dates	15 gm
Tamarind	2 tsp
Coriander	25 gm
Mint leaves	25 gm
Raw mango	25 gm
Black pepper	1 tsp
Pomegranate	25 gm

Method

- In a bowl, add boiled and mashed potato, boiled peas, cumin seed, salt, turmeric powder and coriander powder. Mix it well and make it in a small round shape like patties. In a pan add oil and cook the patties on both sides till golden brown.
- For tamarind chutney, boil the dates and tamarind together. Then bring it to room temperature and crush it into a paste. For mint chutney, grind raw mango, mint, and coriander in a paste. Whiski in the curd.
- Serve the patties with curd, mint chutney, tamarind chutney, black pepper and pomegranate.

Healthy cooking tips

- Sweet potato is very high in fiber and a replacement for potato.
- It can be taken post-workout as its high in carbohydrates and fibers.
- Skim the cream and then use the milk for setting the curd.

SWEET POTATO CHAT

A scrumptious recipe that is filled with traditional chat flavours and healthy too.

Skill level	Easy
Serving size	2

Place of origin	India
Season most suited for consumption	Winter
Rich in nutrients	Calcium, Iron, Fiber, Beta carotene

Know your nutrition

Sweet potato (Shakarkand): It is rich in fiber, a good source of Vitamin A, C B6, potassium, copper and manganese. It also promotes gut health. May have cancer-fighting properties and enhance brain function. It also boosts the immune system.

Sesame seeds (Til): Sesame seed is a good source of calcium that promotes bone health. The magnesium content in seeds also helps to lower cholesterol and triglyceride levels. Vitamin E and other antioxidants in seeds help to maintain blood pressure. Sesame seeds are also a good source of vitamin B. Sesame seeds are low in carbohydrates and high in protein and fiber that helps to control blood sugar level.

Favourable for conditions

Anemia, Bone health, Athletes

Calorie count

Serving Size	Energy (Kcal)	Carbohydrate (gm)	Protein (gm)	Fats (gm)	Calcium (mg)
1	137	20	3.9	3.6	114.5
2	275	40	7.8	7.2	229
Serving Size	Phosphorus (mg)	Total Fiber (mg)	Omega-3 (mg)	Iron (mg)	Beta carotene (mcg)
1	61.5	5.7	59.2	3.3	2669.7
2		11.4	118.4	6.6	5339.4

Ingredients

Sweet potato	100 gms
Pomegranate	25 gm
Mint leaves	25 gm
Mung sprout	15 gm
Til seed	15 gm
Coriander	1 tsp
Salt	¼ tsp
Amchur powder	2 tsp
Cumin powder	1 tsp

Method

- Wash the sweet potato and boil it.
- In a bowl add sweet potato, pomegranate, mint leaves, mung sprout, salt, amchur powder, cumin powder and mix it well.
- Add coriander and til seed and serve.

Healthy cooking tips

- Instead of mung sprout, any other sprout like chana sprout or matki sprout can also be used.
- Sweet potato is very high in fiber and a replacement for potato.
- It can also be used as a thickener.
- Do not roast sweet potato as it increases the dietary AGE (advanced glycation end products). Steam and cook instead.
- It can be consumed post-workout as its high in carbohydrates and high fibers.

2. DOSA

MORINGA DOSA

A nourishing version of the dosa with the incorporation of moringa/drumstick leaves.

Skill level	Easy
Serving size	6
Place of origin	South India, India
Season most suited for consumption	All seasons
Rich in nutrients	Sodium, Potassium, Calcium, Phosphorous, Beta- Carotene

Know your nutrition

Moringa: It reduces inflammation as it is rich in anti-inflammatory compounds. It has antioxidant power since it is rich in vitamin C, quercetin and chlorogenic acid. It helps in treating cancer as it is rich in niazimicin (an anti-cancer agent) that restrains the development of cancer cells. It improves the heart health by effectively reducing cholesterol level. It improves bones health as it is rich in calcium and phosphorous, which increase bone mass and structural strength.

Brown rice: Brown rice is a whole grain and a good source of magnesium, phosphorus, selenium, thiamine, niacin, vitamin B6, and manganese, and the fiber in it helps manage cholesterol, moves waste through the digestive tract, gives satiety, and helps to prevent the formation of blood clots.

Carom seeds (Ajwain): A spice for stomach issues such as indigestion, flatulence, diarrhea and colic. It aids in relieving respiratory ailments. It is used as a cleanser, detox, diuretic and antacid.

Favourable for conditions

Anemia, Pregnancy, Diabetes, Muscle and Bone health

Calorie count

Serving Size	Energy (Kcal)	Carbohydrate (gm)	Total Fiber (mg)	Protein (gm)	Fats (gm)	Omega-3 (mg)
1	200.3	35.8	3.1	5.8	1.5	26.3
6	1201.9	214.8	19.1	34.96	9.5	157.8
Serving Size	Calcium (mg)	Phosphorous (mg)	Beta-carotene (mcg)	Sodium (mg)	Potassium (mg)	Magnesium (mg)
1	23.3	52	660.9	146.6	19.3	12.8
6	140.3	312.5	3965.8	880	1076.2	77.3

Ingredients

Rice	200 gm
Urad dal	100 gm
Moringa (Drumstick leaves)	50 gm
Peanuts	15 gm
Salt	½ tsp
Oil	1 tsp
Carom seeds (Ajwain)	½ tsp

Method

- Soak rice and urad dal for 3 hours. Drain and blend in a blender. Keep aside for 5 hours for it to ferment.
- Make a purée of the moringa leaves and crush the peanuts.
- Add salt, carom seeds, peanuts and the puréed leaves to the fermented batter and mix well.
- Take a tawa/pan, put some oil on it and pour some batter at the center. With a spoon spread the batter on the tawa gently in a circular motion and let it cook for 2-3 minutes, or until golden brown.
- Serve with any sabzi or chutney.

Healthy cooking tips

- It is a versatile vegetable and a great flavouring agent. It contains a good amount of fiber and anti-diabetic properties. Dry roast on a tawa and powder the curry leaves and add in the recipe. It can be added to smoothies and salads.
- Do not strain the rice water away. Use it in other preparations like soups.
- If rice is unprocessed, you can also sprout it to increase its nutritional value.

❧

MULTI-LENTIL DOSA

An authentic crispy dosa recipe with abundance of protein-rich lentils.

Skill level	Moderate
Serving size	5
Place of origin	South India, India
Season most suited for consumption	All seasons
Rich in nutrients	Protein, Calcium, Potassium, Magnesium, Phosphorus

Know your nutrition

Mung gram (Yellow mung dal): It is a plant-based source of protein, ideal for vegetarians and vegans. It is a good source of zinc and vitamin B1. It is light and very easy to digest. It helps in stabilizing blood sugar.

Black gram (urad dal): It is a plant-based source of protein, ideal for vegetarians and vegans. It is a source of zinc and potassium. It aids in digestion and prevents anemia. It improves heart health due to the presence of magnesium, fiber, and potassium.

White rice: White rice is a good source of magnesium, phosphorus, manganese, selenium, iron, folic acid, thiamine, and niacin, and additionally, its low fiber content may help with digestive issues.

Favourable for conditions

Children, Senior Citizens, Digestion, Hypertension, Cardiac Health, Immunity, Stress

Calorie count

Serving Size	Energy (Kcal)	Carbohydrate (gm)	Protein (gm)	Fats (gm)	Calcium (mg)	Folate (mcg)
1	250	44.3	6.9	1	15.3	7.8
5	1249	221.7	34.4	4.8	76.3	38.9

Serving Size	Phosphorus (mg)	Potassium (mg)	Magnesium (mg)	Total Fiber (mg)	Omega-3 (mg)
1	92.8	208.6	23.7	3.3	12.2
5	463.9	1042.8	118.3	16.4	61

Ingredients

Rice	1 cup
Ajwain seeds	1 tsp
Mint powder	1 tsp
Mungdal	½ cup
Urad dal	½ cup
Turmeric powder	½ tsp
Oil	1 tbsp
Salt	½ tsp
Water	To grind

Method

- Wash and soak the rice and the dals for 4–6 hours or overnight.
- After the rice and lentils are soaked, drain the water. Grind

the lentils with little water until smooth.

- Add all spices and salt and mix well.
- Heat a tawa and once it is hot smear it with some oil.
- Pour a ladle of batter in the center of the tawa and spread it quickly into a thin large circle.
- Pour a tsp of oil around the edges and cook on medium heat until the dosa is crisp and golden. Serve with coconut chutney or any other chutney of your choice.

Healthy cooking tips

- Soak the dals at least for 6–8 hours.
- Wash well and discard the water. Discarding water may reduce bloating and can also reduce uric acid levels.
- Prefer eating chana and urad dal only in the afternoon, as consumed in the night may cause bloating and flatulence.
- Do not add soda to it whilst cooking.
- Ajwain is great for digestion and can be used effectively as post-meal mukhwas and to relief bloating or flatulence. Ajwain water is advised to be consumed post meals or ajwain could even be consumed raw.

3. FRUIT- OR VEGETABLE-BASED SNACKS

FRUIT PLATE

An everyday recipe with amalgamation of vibrant fruits and goodness of water chestnuts.

Skill level	Easy
Serving size	2
Place of origin	India
Season most suited for consumption	Monsoon
Rich in nutrients	Fiber, Calcium, Magnesium, Potassium, Vitamin C

Know your nutrition

Water chestnuts: These contain polyphenols and a good amount of calcium aiding in muscle contractions and enhancing the bone mineral density. They have plenty of fiber and may help promote bowel movements, reduce blood cholesterol levels, regulate blood sugar levels and keep the gut healthy.

Apple: Apples are rich in pectin and soluble as well as insoluble fibers relieving digestive disorders. It improves heart health and cholesterol levels because of the presence of quercetin and micro-minerals. It has a low glycemic index and hence provides satiety.

Strawberry: The bioactive component present in strawberry is Anthocyanin, known for its anti-oxidative properties, which protects the body from carcinogens (cancer-causing radicals) and is anti-inflammatory in nature, thus anti-aging too. The overall presence of anti-oxidants and vitamin C benefits cardiovascular health.

Favourable for conditions

Pregnancy, Bone health, Hypertension, Cardiac Health, Immunity, Stress

Calorie count

Serving Size	Energy (Kcal)	Carbohydrate (gm)	Protein (gm)	Fats (gm)	Calcium (mg)	Phosphorus (mg)
1	163	35.8	1.3	1.5	35.3	32.8
2	326	71.7	2.6	3	70.6	65.6
Serving Size	Potassium (mg)	Magnesium (mg)	Total Fiber (mg)	Omega-3 (mg)	Vitamin C (mg)	
1	179	15.1	5	24.8	15.3	
2	358	30.2	10.1	49.6	30.6	

Ingredients

Apple	½ cup
Water chestnut	½ cup
Strawberry	4–5
Dates	3–4
Honey	1 tbsp
Chia seeds	2 tsp
Ginger	1 inch

Method

- Cut apples, strawberry, water chestnut and dates into small pieces add grated ginger and mix well.
- Then add honey and chia seeds on it and serve.

Healthy cooking tips

- Apple should be consumed with the skin. Place it in water warm water for a few minutes to remove the outer waxy layer; store them after cutting, apply some lime over it to avoid discolouration.
- Water chestnut can be eaten raw after peeling it or can cook it and then peel and eat it.
- Strawberry is rich in vitamin C and has a lot of cancer fighting properties, beneficial for diabetic patients and can be made into a juice or incorporated into smoothie, yogurt, salads or ice-cream.

BEETROOT KHANDVI

A vibrant version of classic Gujarati khandvi recipe with the goodness of beetroot.

Skill level	Moderate
Serving size	2
Place of origin	Gujarat, India
Season most suited for consumption	All seasons
Rich in nutrients	Calcium, Vitamin B12, Potassium, Fiber, Folate, Iron

Know your nutrition

Bengal Gram (Herbera/Black chickpea): It is a plant-based source of protein, ideal for vegetarians and vegans. It is a source of iron, folate and copper, and provides satiety and energy. It stabilizes blood sugar, which prevents diabetes. They also contain phytochemicals called saponins that act as antioxidants.

Beetroot (Beet): It can lower blood sugar and also improve oxygen use, stamina, and exercise performance. The high concentration of nitrates enhance athletic performance by improving oxygen use and boosting energy. It may help fight inflammation and improve digestive health and brain health.

Favourable for conditions

Weight Loss, Senior Citizens, Children, Adolescents, Bone, and Muscle health

Calorie count

Serving Size	Energy (Kcal)	Carbohydrate (gm)	Protein (gm)	Fats (gm)	Calcium (mg)	Phosphorus (mg)
1	325	23.5	8.3	12.3	96.9	100.3
2	162	11.8	4.2	6.2	48.5	50.2

Serving Size	Total Fiber (mg)	Omega-3 (mg)	Total folate (mcg)	Vitamin A (mcg)	Potassium (mg)	
1	7.7	33	99.8	115.7	493.4	
2	3.9	16.5	49.9	57.9	246.7	

Ingredients

Beetroot	50 gm
Besan	30 gm
Curd	50 gm
Ginger paste	1 tsp
Coriander leaves	2 tsp
Grated fresh coconut	3 tbsp
Curry leaves	4–5
Filtered Rice bran oil	2 tsp

Method

- Boil beetroot in a small pot, let it cool and make a purée.
- Add besan, beetroot purée, curd in a bowl and mix into a smooth paste.
- Add coconut and coriander leaves in another bowl and mix it.
- Add the besan mixture in a pan with little oil and ginger paste and stir it into a thick paste.
- When it is thickened immediately spread it on a steel plate and sprinkle coconut mixture over it.
- Take oil in a small bowl and let it heat for some time. Add curry leaves and pour that on the besan mixture sheet once it is cooled.
- Cut the sheets into pieces, roll it, and serve hot.

Healthy cooking tips

- To retain nutrients and colour, boil, or steam without peeling first. Doing this will ensure that the skin easily comes off under cold water.

- For the best flavour, bake the beetroots instead of boiling or steaming. Wrap them in aluminum foil to avoid staining.

✿

LAAL BHOPLYA CHE GHARGE

An appeasing Maharashtrian sweet delight made of pumpkin.

Skill level	Easy
Serving size	4
Place of origin	Maharashtra, India
Season most suited for consumption	Winter
Rich in nutrients	Vitamin A, Thiamin.

Know your nutrition

Pumpkin: Pumpkin has antioxidant such as beta carotene that protects the body from free radicals. It is also rich in vitamin A that helps in improving eyesight and also a good source of vitamin C, vitamin E, iron, potassium, and folate. It has a high content of water and also has high amounts of fiber that provides satiety and decreases digestion-related problems. Augments immunity and promotes eye health.

Fennel seeds (Saunf): It has applications for strengthening agni without aggravating pitta curing issues of the digestive system, bones, joints, allergies and cold pain. It significantly decreases low-density lipoprotein—bad cholesterol levels, thus reducing inflammations and peroxidative damage, preventing risks of degenerative diseases, boosting immunity and metabolism.

Nutmeg (Jaifhal): It helps to stop diarrhea (in low dose), detoxify the body, and stimulate the brain. It has antioxidant, antimicrobial and antifungal properties. However, consuming too much nutmeg results in a sudden attack, irregular heart palpitations and vomiting.

Favourable for conditions

Athletes, Children, Eyes health

Calorie count

Serving Size	Energy (Kcal)	Carbohydrate (gm)	Total Fiber (mg)	Protein (gm)	Fats (gm)	Omega-3 (mg)
1	194	43.5	0.8	6.6	1	3.3
4	777	174	3.3	6	4.1	13.4

Serving Size	Calcium (mg)	Potassium (mg)	Sodium (mg)	Magnesium (mg)	Beta-carotene (mcg)	Iron (mcg)
1	46.8	226.3	444.7	25.7	9.4	2.2
4	187.4	905.4	1779	103	37.8	9.1

Ingredients

Pumpkin grated	50 gm
Whole wheat flour	30 gm
Jaggery	10 tbsp
Oil	2 gm
Nutmeg, grated	2 gm
Saunf	5 gm
Himalayan pink salt	2 gms

Method

- Mix grated pumpkin and jaggery, salt nutmeg and saunf on a hot pan.
- Add semolina, wheat flour, 1 tbsp hot oil and mix well.
- Knead to a firm dough (use little water if required or more flour if it is too sticky).
- Make small balls from the dough and roll out into round shape.

- Grease the pan, roast them like chapati till they turn light brown.
- Drain on an absorbent paper.

Healthy cooking tips

- Avoid deep-frying to retain the health benefits, unlike the traditional recipe.

RAW BANANA TIKKIS

Finger-licking tikkis enriched with raw banana and nutritious vegetables.

Skill level	Moderate
Serving size	4
Place of origin	India
Season most suited for consumption	All seasons
Rich in nutrients	Vitamin C, A, Fiber, Potassium

Know your nutrition

Raw banana: Raw bananas contain high amount of resistant starch and pectin, which have been linked to several health benefits like improved blood sugar control and better digestive health. It has a high potassium content that would support muscle contractions.

Peanut/groundnut (Mungfali): Peanuts are high in energy. It improves heart health and prevents gallstones. It contains niacin that protects against Alzheimer's disease and cognitive decline. It contains a good amount of folate, which is good for pregnant women. The magnesium content of peanuts helps to reduce the inflammation.

Carrot (Gajar): They are a good source of Vitamin A, biotin, Vitamin K, potassium, and Vitamin B6. Carrots improve eyesight and immune function, provides satiety, and prevents constipation. It also reduces the risk of cancer.

Favourable for conditions

Digestion, Children, Constipation, Hypertension, Cardiac Health

Calorie count

Serving Size	Phosphorus (mg)	Energy (Kcal)	Carbohydrate (gm)	Protein (gm)	Fats (gm)	Calcium (mg)
1	16.3	119	5.7	1.4	10.1	11.6
4	65.2	477	22.7	5.6	40.3	46.6
Serving Size	Potassium (mg)	Sodium (mg)	Total Fiber (mg)	Omega-3 (mg)	Vitamin A (mcg)	Folate (mcg)
1	129.3	449.7	1.8	7	70.1	16.1
4	517.1	1799.1	7.3	27.9	280.3	64.5

Ingredients

Banana, raw, boiled and grated	1 (50 g)
Beetroot, boiled and grated	1 (75 g)
Carrot, boiled and grated	½ (30 g)
Coconut, freshly grated	2 tbsp
Ginger, grated	1 inch
Coriander powder	½ tsp
Peanut, roasted	1 tbsp
Cumin powder	½ tsp
Ajwain seeds	1 tsp
Groundnut oil	2 tbsp
Salt	½ tsp

Method

- Boil the carrot, beetroot, and pressure cook banana for 2 whistles and set aside. Once cool, grate them.

- In a bowl add oil coconut, ginger, ajwain, cumin, coriander, and peanut then mix the vegetables, including salt, and shape into tikkis.
- Shallow fry the tikkis in a pan on both sides until light brown in colour; enjoy with chutney of your choice.

Healthy cooking tips

- Slightly raw banana or elaichi banana can be consumed by people who want to lose weight or are diabetes patients, since it contains less sugar compared to ripe bananas.
- Raw beetroot has a lower glycemic index compared to cooked beetroot and is beneficial for diabetic patients. Beetroot juice helps to reduce blood pressure, improves metabolism, and exercise stamina; beetroot can be added to salads, smoothies, soups, rotis, rice.

๙

ROASTED MAKHANA

A healthy calcium-rich snack with the nutty flavour.

Skill level	Easy
Serving size	2
Place of origin	India
Season most suited for consumption	All seasons
Rich in nutrients	Calcium

Know your nutrition

Makhana has inflammatory properties. It's good for our spleen health and also maintains blood pressure. It is beneficial for arthritis patients.

Favourable for conditions

Weight loss, Diabetes, Athletes, Children, Adolescents, Pregnancy, Bone and Muscle health

Calorie count

Serving size	Energy (Kcal)	Carbohydrates (gm)	Protein (gm)	Fats (gm)	Omega-3 (mg)
1	59	8.8	1	2	2.2
2	118	17.6	2	4	4.4
Serving size	Calcium gm	Phosphorus gm	Iron gm		
1	2.3	6.3	0.3		
2	4.7	12.7	0.7		

Ingredients

Makhana (Foxnuts)	3 cups
Turmeric powder (Haldi)	¼ tsp
Rock salt	½ tsp
Oil or ghee	1 tsp

Method

- Heat oil in a pan or kadhai.
- Add the makhana and roast for a good 5 minutes on a low flame till they become crisp and crunchy.
- Keep on stirring in between.
- Add turmeric powder and salt.
- Toss the whole mixture well.

Healthy cooking tips

- Foxnuts are great for weight loss. They are an ideal tiffin snack and travel food.

4. UPMA/DALIA

CHAWAL NU KHICHU

Stimulating Gujarati cuisine snack with high nutritional value.

Skill level	Moderate
Serving size	2
Place of origin	Gujarat, India
Season most suited for consumption	Monsoon, Autumn, Winter
Rich in nutrients	Calcium

Know your nutrition

Rice flour: Rice flour is a good source of magnesium, phosphorus, manganese, selenium, iron, folic acid, thiamine, and niacin, and additionally, its low fiber content may help with digestive issues.

Cow's ghee: It has a neutral taste. It contains medium and short-chain fatty acids that help to improve digestion and reduce bowel problems and also help boost immunity. It contains vitamin K that helps to reduce arthritis and enhances bone health. It also helps in the proper functioning of the heart and boosts the good cholesterol level. It contains omega-6 fatty acid that helps to reduce insulin resistance and lowers blood sugar levels. It also helps in healing external wounds and improves eye health.

Favourable for conditions

Bone health, High blood pressure, Children, Adolescents

Calorie count

Serving Size	Energy (Kcal)	Carbohydrate (gm)	Protein (gm)	Fats (gm)
1	175	22.6	5.7	5.8
2	350	45.2	11.4	11.6

Serving Size	Calcium (mg)	Phosphorus (mg)	Total Fiber (mg)	Omega-3 (mg)
1	110	35.5	3.6	10
2	220	71	7.2	20

Ingredients

Rice flour	60 gm
Til seed	15 gm
Cumin seed	½ tsp
Salt	¼ tsp
Ghee	¼ tsp

Method

- In a vessel add water along with cumin seed.
- After 2 minutes very slowly add the rice flour and keep stirring continuously so that no lumps are formed.
- Add salt and stir for another 2 minutes till a thick paste is achieved.
- Pour it in a bowl and add ghee and til seeds.

Healthy cooking tips

- While adding the flour keep stirring continuously so that lumps are not formed.
- Keep stirring until it forms a dough and doesn't stick to the vessel.
- Add the boiling water carefully.
- One can also use wheat flour as an alternative.
- One can also add coriander and ajwain seed to enhance the flavour of the dish.

OATS UPMA

A wholesome version of authentic upma with the richness of oats and vegetables.

Skill level	Easy
Serving size	2
Place of origin	India
Season most suited for consumption	All seasons
Rich in nutrients	Manganese, Phosphorous, Copper, Vitamin B, Iron, Selenium, Fiber

Know your nutrition

Whole oats are rich in antioxidants, and contain a powerful soluble fiber called Beta-Glucan. It can lower cholesterol levels and protect LDL cholesterol from damage. Oats can improve blood sugar control.

Favourable for conditions

Weight Loss, Diabetes, Heart Health, Children, Adolescents, Pregnancy, Bone and Muscle health

Calorie count

Serving Size	Energy (Kcal)	Carbohydrate (gm)	Protein (gm)	Fats (gm)	Calcium (mg)	Vitamin A (mcg)
1	170	24.1	3.2	3	39.5	258.5
2	341	48.3	6.4	6	79	517

Serving Size	Phosphorus (mg)	Total Fiber (mg)	Omega-3 (mg)	Total Folate (mcg)	Potassium (mg)	
1	75.1	3.9	14	18.5	14	
2	150.2	7.7	28.1	37	28.1	

Ingredients

Oats	60 gm
Ghee	1 tsp
Carrot	50 gm
Beans	25 gm
Tomato	25 gm
Sweet corn	50 gm
Curry leaves	1-2
Cumin seeds	1-2
Ajwain	1 tsp
Lemon juice	¼ tsp
Salt	½ tsp

Method

- In a pan, sauté oats for few minutes, once they are little crispy. Remove from heat and let it cool down.
- In a pan, add carrot, beans, tomato, and sweet corn and let them cook for 10-15 minutes with lid closed.
- In a separate pan, add ghee, cumin seeds, curry leaves, and ajwain. Add the cooked veggies, oats, and salt in the pan, mix well, and let it cook for 5-10 minutes.
- Add water if needed.
- Once cooked remove from the heat and add lemon juice to the mixture, mix well.
- Serve hot.

Healthy cooking tips

- Use steel-cut rolled oats and not processed oats or instant oats.

PONKH UPMA

Ponkh are tender jowar seeds, a seasonal Gujarat speciality

Skill level	Moderate
Serving size	3
Place of origin	Gujarat, India
Season most suited for consumption	Autumn, Winter
Rich in nutrients	Beta carotene, Calcium, Potassium, Sodium

Know your nutrition

Ponkh: Ponkh is very high in fiber with a high protein level as well. The fiber helps in slow release of sugar in the blood and helps control cholesterol levels. Ponkh is gluten-free, an attractive alternative for those who have wheat allergy. It also is packed with a few minerals like iron, magnesium, phosphorus, and zinc.

Coconut (Nariyal): Coconut is low in carbohydrates and high in fiber, which helps stabilize blood sugar. Coconut has an anti-diabetic effect due to its arginine content. It is high in antioxident, which also prevents oxidative damage.

Coriander leaves: Coriander reduces cholesterol deposition by lowering cholesterol levels and blood sugar. It is good for digestion as it contains high insoluble fiber and reduces Urinary Tract Infection. It is rich in vitamin C, hence possesses antioxidant activity.

Favourable for conditions

Gluten-free, Children, Senior Citizens, Pregnancy, Lactation, Digestion, Athletes, Anemia

Calorie count

Serving Size	Energy (Kcal)	Carbohydrate (gm)	Protein (gm)	Fats (gm)	Calcium (mg)	Phosphorus (mg)
1	166	23.6	3.3	5.3	31.4	62.2
3	489	70.9	9.8	94.2	18.8	186.8

Serving Size	Total Fiber (mg)	Omega-3 (mg)	Potassium (mg)	Sodium (mg)	Beta-Carotene (mcg)	
1	3	91.7	146.3	579.8	106.2	
3	8.9	275	438.9	1739.7	318.6	

Ingredients:

Ponkh	2 cups
Oil	2 tsp
Mustard seeds	½ tbsp
Cumin seeds	¼ tbsp
Curry leaves	8 to 10
Grated coconut	2 tbsp
Chopped coriander	1/3 tsp
Salt	as required

Method

- First rinse ponkh in a fine strainer or colander.
- Heat oil in a pan.
- Add mustard seeds and let them crackle.
- When the mustard seed begins to crackle, add cumin seeds. Let the cumin seeds splutter.
- Then add 8 to 10 chopped curry leaves.
- Mix well and sauté on low to medium flame.
- Add the tender ponkh.
- Season with salt as per taste.
- Mix well and sauté for a couple of minutes or until the grains are cooked. Stir often when sautéing.
- Lastly, add grated coconut and mix well.

- Remove from the flame, add chopped coriander leaves, mix well and serve.

Healthy cooking tips:

- Heat the oil thoroughly before adding seasoning or vegetables.
- Coconut itself contains a good amount of oil so while using coconut use less oil in the recipes.

❦

SAVOURY DALIA

A delicious dalia recipe that fulfils the hunger cravings.

Skill level	Easy
Serving size	4
Place of origin	India
Season most suited for consumption	All seasons
Rich in nutrients	Phosphorus, calcium, folic acid

Know your nutrition:

Dalia (broken wheat): Dalia is a good source of magnesium. High fiber helps in controlling the levels of cholesterol, which reduces the risk of strokes. It is rich in vitamins and fiber. Fiber-rich foods like bulgur may reduce chronic disease risk, also aids in weight loss, improves digestion and gut health.

Sesame seed: Sesame seed is a good source of calcium that promotes bone health. Magnesium content in seeds also helps to lower cholesterol and triglycerides levels. Vitamin E and other antioxidants in seeds help to maintain blood pressure. Sesame seeds are also a good source of vitamin B. Sesame seeds are low in carbohydrates and high in protein and fiber that helps to control blood sugar levels.

Favourable for conditions

Weight loss, Diabetes, Anemia, Cardiac Health, Women's health, PCOS, Pregnancy, Lactation.

Calorie count

Serving Size	Energy (Kcal)	Carbohydrate (gm)	Protein (gm)	Fats (gm)	Calcium (mg)
1	275	35.5	8	9.2	86.8
4	1099	141.9	32.1	36.8	347.1
Serving Size	Phosphorus (mg)	Total Fiber (mg)	Omega-3 (mg)	Folic acid (mcg)	
1	124.5	5.4	17.5	71	
4	498	21.8	69.9	284.2	

Ingredients

Cooked dalia	2 cup
Groundnut	¼ cup
Roasted and ground sesame seeds	2 tbsp
Refined vegetable oil	1 tsp
Mustard Seeds	¼ tsp
Turmeric powder	¼ tsp
Curry leaves	Few
Lime	½
Salt	½ tsp

Method

- Mix cooked dalia, tamarind paste, ground sesame seeds and salt in a bowl. Take care that all ingredients are mixed well and evenly.
- In a non-stick pan, heat some oil, sputter mustard seeds, add groundnut and roast.
- Once done, add curry leaves and turmeric powder and mix.
- Add all the ingredients mixed earlier and sauté for a minute.

- Sprinkle lime juice and mix well.
- Serve hot with curd.

Healthy cooking tips

- The alternative for dalia can be quinoa or khus khus.

❦

SEMIYA UPMA

South Indian version of upma that is wholesome and has an umami flavour.

Skill level	Moderate
Serving size	2
Place of origin	South India, India
Season most suited for consumption	All seasons
Rich in nutrients	Protein, Zinc, Potassium, Vitamin C, Vitamin K

Know your nutrition

Wheat: Wheat is important because it is high in fiber, vitamins, antioxidants and minerals. It lowers the risk of diabetes, heart disease and high blood pressure. It is known for controlling obesity.

Black gram (Urad dal): It is a plant-based source of protein, ideal for vegetarians and vegans. It is a source of zinc and potassium. It aids in digestion and prevents Anemia. It improves heart health due to the presence of magnesium, fiber and potassium.

Coriander (Dhania): It reduces cholesterol deposition by lowering cholesterol levels and blood sugar. It is good for digestion as it contains high insoluble fiber and reduces Urinary Tract Infection. It is rich in vitamin C hence possesses antioxidant activity and vitamin K. It can ease muscle spasms and flatulence.

Favourable for conditions

Anemia, Heart disease, Urinary tract infection, High cholesterol

Calorie count

Serving Size	Energy (Kcal)	Carbohydrate (gm)	Protein (gm)	Fats (gm)	Calcium (mg)	Phosphorus (mg)	Total Fiber (mg)	Omega-3 (mg)
1	218	36.8	4.2	4.6	21.9	35.7	3.4	46.6
2	437	73.7	8.3	9.3	43.8	71.4	6.7	93.2

Ingredients

Broken semiya	1 cup
Mustard seeds	½ tsp
Urad dal	1 tsp
Cumin seeds	½ tsp
Finely chopped ginger	½ tsp
Curry leaves	1 tsp
Chopped coriander	2 tbsp
Hing	1 tsp
Oil	1 tbsp
Salt	1 tsp

Method

- Roast the broken semiya in a kadhai till it turns golden.
- Take a pan, add oil, mustard seeds, cumin seeds, urad dal. Mix well and fry till the urad dal turns golden.
- Add curry leaves, ginger, hang and sauté. Now add water, salt and let the mixture come to a boil.
- Add the roasted semiya, cook till it becomes soft and all the water is absorbed. Switch off the flame and serve the semiya upma garnished with corianders leave along with some lemon.

Healthy cooking tips

- Squeeze the lemon on top while serving to increase the vitamin C content.
- It can also include vegetables such as carrot, green peas, etc.
- Roast the spices on a medium flame.
- Do not overcook the semiya.
- Many people discard the curry leaf from dals and vegetables. Dry roast them on a tawa and powder the curry leaves and add up in the recipe.

5. UTTAPAM

MULTIGRAIN UTTAPAM

South Indian breakfast pancake, which has a blend of multi-grains and lentils with the natural sweetness of coconut.

Skill level	Moderate
Serving size	5
Place of origin	Tamil Nadu, India
Season most suited for consumption	All seasons
Rich in nutrients	Beta-carotene, Calcium, Phosphorous, Magnesium, Fiber, Protein, Phosphorous, Beta-Glucan

Know your nutrition

Black gram (Urad dal): It is a plant-based source of protein, ideal for vegetarians and vegans. It is a source of zinc and potassium. It aids in digestion and prevents anemia. It improves heart health due to the presence of magnesium, fiber, and potassium.

Brown rice: Brown rice is a wholegrain and a good source of magnesium, phosphorus, selenium, thiamine, niacin, vitamin B6, and manganese. The fiber in it helps manage cholesterol; moves waste through the digestive tract, gives satiety, and helps to prevent blood formation.

Oats: Whole oats are rich in antioxidants, and contain a powerful soluble fiber called beta-glucan. They can lower cholesterol levels and protect LDL cholesterol from damage. Oats can improve blood sugar levels.

Favourable for conditions

Diabetes, Weight loss, Senior citizens

Calorie count

Serving Size	Energy (Kcal)	Carbohydrate (gm)	Total Fiber (mg)	Protein (gm)	Fats (gm)	Magnesium (mg)
1	218	31.2	6	7.8	4.4	16.6
5	1093	156.3	28	39	22	83.2
Serving Size	Omega-3 (mg)	Calcium (mg)	Potassium (mg)	Beta-carotene (mg)	Phosphorous (mg)	
1	18.5	20.7	294	94	83.25	
5	93	103	1470.8	470.4	435.6	

Ingredients

Rice	50 gm
Urad dal	100 gm
Oats	50 gm
Mung dal	50 gm
Tomatoes	100 gms
Cabbage	100 gms (chopped)
Coconut	50 gms
Pepper	A pinch
Salt	½ tsp

Method

- Wash and soak the grains for 6-8 hours.
- Blend them together and add salt. Keep aside for ½ hour. (You can add curd at this step).
- Chop tomatoes and cabbage and add to the mixer along with a pinch of pepper powder and desiccated coconut.
- Take a pan or tawa, put some oil in it and pour the batter in the center and spread it in an 8-10 cm diameter or any size and thickness of your choice. Cook for 2-3 minutes or until golden brown.
- Serve with coconut chutney or have it plain.

Healthy cooking tips

- Consume the urad only in the afternoon.
- Soak it overnight and discard the water because the water will have a white frothy layer that creates flatulence. Wash well and cook it.
- Use steel-cut rolled oats and not processed oats or instant oats.
- Soak oats in water for 10 minutes and then use them in preparations.

SPINACH UTTAPAM

A scrumptious South Indian pancake that offers the goodness of spinach and a blend of essential nutrie.

Skill level	Moderate
Serving size	3
Place of origin	South India, India
Season most suited for consumption	All seasons
Rich in nutrients	Potassium, Magnesium, Calcium, Iron, Folate, Vitamin A, C

Know your nutrition

Spinach (palak): It is rich in fiber that induces satiety and also aids in weight loss. It helps to reduce the risk of cancer as it contains anticancer agents and antioxidants such as flavonoids, vitamin C, E and carotenoids, improve eyesight as it is rich in lutein and zeaxanthin which protect the eyes and reverse blindness. It is a good source of calcium, magnesium, potassium, iron, and folate. It is also useful to reduce GI disorders as it is rich in fiber.

Cumin seeds (Jeera): Ayurveda proves the benefits of cumin in the GI, reproductive, nervous and immune systems. It is antioxidant, antimicrobial and chemoprotective. It is also anti-diabetic, antiseptic, relieves flatulence, and is a metabolic stimulator.

Favourable for conditions

Anemia, Diabetes, Hypertension, Cardiac Health, Immunity, Stress

Calorie count

Serving Size	Energy (Kcal)	Carbohydrate (gm)	Protein (gm)	Fats (gm)	Calcium (mg)	Phosphorus (mg)	Iron (mg)
1	232	30.2	6.5	5.8	28.3	93.5	0.7
3	696	90.7	19.4	17.5	84.8	280.4	2.2

Serving Size	Potassium (mg)	Magnesium (mg)	Total Fiber (mg)	Omega-3 (mg)	Vitamin A (mcg)	Vitamin C (mg)	Folate (mcg)
1	179	9.6	2.9	17.5	87.8	1.1	17.6
3	537	28.7	8.6	52.5	263.5	3.4	52.9

Ingredients

Urad sprouts	½ cup
Oats powder	1 cup
Carrot, grated	1 tbsp
Tomato, chopped	1 (30 g)

Spinach	½ cup purée
Cumin powder	½ tsp
Amchur powder	¼ tsp
Coriander powder	1 tsp
Salt	¼ tsp
Oil	For greasing

Method

- Grind the sprouts and spinach separately into a smooth paste and transfer in a bowl. Add oats powder, coriander powder, cumin powder, salt, amchur powder, and mix well.
- In a pan, put ghee and spread little thick batter. Add tomato and carrot on it and let it cook. Then flip it and let it cook until it turns slightly brown.
- Transfer it on a plate and serve it with a chutney of your choice.

Healthy cooking tips

- Spinach should be washed well and make sure that it does not have worms. Spinach is a mild-flavoured, healthy green that makes for a powerful ingredient in salads, smoothies, soups, pastas, sandwiches, rotis and rice.
- Wash the carrots well and use it along with skin; cooking carrots enhances their lycopene content and increases vitamin A availability.
- Soak it overnight and discard the water because the water above will have a white frothy layer that needs to discard because it creates lots of flatulence. Consume it only in the afternoon.

6. VEGETABLE SNACKS

VEGETABLE BUCKWHEAT

A comfort bowl of energetic vegetables with an abundance of essential nutrients, vitamins, minerals and fiber.

Skill level	Moderate
Serving size	2
Place of origin	India
Season most suited for consumption	All seasons
Rich in nutrients	Beta carotene, Vitamin B9

Know your nutrition

Buckwheat (Kuttu): Buckwheat is rich in fiber, which supports the intestines in digesting food efficiently and helps food move through the digestive tract. It may also have other benefits, such as encouraging weight loss and preventing cardiovascular disease. Buckwheat is a source of complex carbohydrates, and helps manage their blood glucose levels.

Broccoli: Helps in reducing cholesterol and lowers blood pressure. It also reduces the risk of cancer. Broccoli is a good source of several vitamins and minerals such as vitamin A, C, B9, and zinc. It also has a good content of beta-carotene and lutein that protects the skin and also helps in relieving inflammation.

Favourable for conditions

Gluten-free, Weight loss, Diabetes

Calorie count

Serving Size	Energy (Kcal)	Carbohydrate (gm)	Protein (gm)	Fats (gm)	Calcium (mg)
1	139	15.9	3.5	5.9	34
2	278	31.8	7.0	11.8	68

Serving Size	Phosphorus (mg)	Total Fiber (mg)	Omega-3 (mg)	Beta carotene (mcg)	Vitamin B9 (mcg)
1	58.2	3.2	15.0	18.9	614.3
2	116.4	6.4	30.0	37.8	1228.6

Ingredients

Buckwheat	30 gm
Peanut	15 gm
Carrot	25 gm
Broccoli	25 gm
Corn	25 gm
Tomatoes	25 gm
Cumin seeds	1 tsp
Curry leaves	3-4
Turmeric powder	2 tsp
Coriander powder	1 tsp
Salt	¼ tsp
Oil	1 tsp

Method

- Boil water in a vessel. In another pan add oil, cumin seeds, curry leaves and peanuts. After 15 seconds, add carrot, broccoli and corn, and sauté for 2-3 min.
- Add tomatoes and sauté for 1 minute. Add the buckwheat and sauté for another 4-5 minutes.
- Then add boiled water along with salt, turmeric powder, and coriander powder and mix it well till water evaporates.
- Serve it in a bowl and garnish with coriander.

Healthy cooking tips

- Buckwheat can be used in making pulao or handvo.
- Healthier alternative to rice as buckwheat is richer in fiber than rice.

- Other vegetables like carrot and beans can also be added. Do not wash vegetables after chopping them. Wash them and then chop the vegetables.
- Sprouted peanuts or boiled peanuts can be used.
- Peanut itself contains a good amount of fat so while using peanut use less oil in the recipes.

7. STEAMED SNACKS

KOTHAMBIR WADI

Maharashtrian delicious crispy snack with the goodness of besan and spinach.

Skill level	Easy
Serving Size	3
Place of origin	Maharashtra, India
Season most suited for Consumption	All seasons
Rich in nutrients	Fiber, Phosphorus, Omega-3 fatty acid

Know your nutrition

Coriander: It reduces cholesterol deposition and blood sugar. It is good for digestion as it contains high insoluble fiber and reduces Urinary Tract Infection. It is rich in vitamin C hence possesses antioxidant activity and vitamin K. It can ease muscle spasms and flatulence.

Sesame seeds: Sesame seed is a good source of calcium that promotes bone health. The magnesium content in seeds also helps to lower cholesterol and triglyceride levels. Vitamin E and other antioxidants in seeds help to maintain blood pressure. Sesame seeds are also a good source of vitamin B. Sesame seeds are low in carbohydrates, high in protein and fiber that helps to control blood sugar levels.

Favourable for conditions

Diabetes, Urinary Tract Infection, Bone health

Calorie count

Serving Size	Energy (Kcal)	Carbohydrate (gm)	Protein (gm)	Fats (gm)	Calcium (mg)
1	190	19.5	7.4	4.7	36.8
3	569	58.7	22.4	14.1	110.6

Serving Size	Phosphorus (mg)	Total Fiber (mg)	Omega-3 (mg)	Potassium (mg)	Beta-Carotene (mcg)
1	69.2	4.4	20	292	331.2
3	207.7	13.4	60.1	875.8	993.8

Ingredients

Besan (Gram flour)	1 cup
Coriander leaves	2 cups
White sesame seeds (roasted)	1 tsp
Asafoetida (Hing)	¼ tsp
Turmeric powder	¼ tsp
Peanut powder (roasted)	1/4 cup
Salt	1 tsp
Oil	2 tsp

Method

- Take a bowl and mix besan, coriander leaves, sesame seeds, salt, turmeric powder, hing, and crushed peanut powder.
- Add water and mix the ingredients into a consistent batter.
- Heat a kadhai, heat 2 tsp of oil, and pour the mixture in it. Steam the batter for 15 mins on high flame, and check whether it is cooked properly.

- Cool it, cut it and add baghar/tadka to it. It can be fried in an air fryer.
- Serve with sauces or chutneys

Healthy cooking tips

- Ensure that the coriander leaves are completely dried before mixing them with the besan, as this is necessary to prevent lumpy dough.
- Use the air fryer technique as it uses minimal or no oil at all. If you do not have an air fryer then steam it on a hot tawa with a lid over it.

❧

PATRA

Delectable tangy Gujarati recipe with the nutritive goodness of colocasia leaves, gram flour and functional superfoods.

Skill level	Moderate
Serving size	3
Place of origin	Gujarat
Season most suited for consumption	All seasons
Rich in nutrients	Magnesium, Potassium, Phosphorus, Iron, Vitamin C, Calcium

Know your nutrition

Colocasia: It helps reduce blood pressure and maintains bone health as it is rich in minerals such as calcium. It has anticoagulant properties, is rich in fiber which aids in weight loss and gives satiety. It is a rich source of beta-carotene, vitamins B and C, iron, potassium, phosphorus and magnesium.

Bengal Gram (Herbera/Black chickpea): It is a plant-based source of protein, ideal for vegetarians and vegans. It is a source of iron, folate and copper and provides satiety and energy. It stabilizes blood sugar, which prevents diabetes. It also contains phytochemicals called saponins which act as antioxidants.

Mustard seeds (Rai): It relieves flatulence, diarrhea, parasite and worm infections, liver diseases, cardiovascular disorders, fevers and regulates immunity. It has antimicrobial, antiseptic and anti-inflammatory properties.

Favourable for conditions

Obesity, Diabetes, Cardiovascular Health

Calorie count

Serving Size	Energy (Kcal)	Carbohydrate (gm)	Protein (gm)	Fats (gm)	Calcium (mg)	Phosphorus (mg)
1	25	19.2	6	2.5	36.5	60.6
3	76	57.7	18.1	7.4	109.4	181.8
Serving Size	Iron (mg)	Potassium (mg)	Magnesium (mg)	Total Fiber (mg)	Omega-3 (mg)	Vitamin C (mg)
1	1	289.5	27.1	4.8	54.4	1.9
3	3.1	868.4	81.4	14.3	163.2	5.6

Ingredients

Colocasia leaves	3 medium size
Coconut flakes	1 tsp
Coriander leaves	1 tbsp

For besan mixture:

| Besan flour | 1 cup |
| Turmeric powder | ½ tsp |

Cumin powder	½ tsp
Garam masala	½ tsp
Water	As required
Salt	To taste
Hing	¼ tsp

For tempering:

Mustard seeds	½ tsp
Oil	1 tsp
Sesame seeds	½ tsp

Method

- In a bowl, add besan, hing, turmeric powder, cumin powder, garam masala, salt and water and make a slightly thick paste. Take colocasia leaves and spread that paste and roll it. Steam the roll for 5-7 minutes.
- In a pan, prepare tempering of mustard and sesame seeds in oil. Cut the roll into slices and put the tempering on it. Garnish coconut flakes and coriander leaves on it and serve with any chutney of choice.

Healthy cooking tips

Cook colocasia well. Otherwise, it may cause mouth rashes. Also, remove the thick vein from the center of the leaf. Colocasia cooks well when the leaves are tender.

8. APPAM

BANANA APPAM

Delectable traditional South Indian recipe with the goodness of banana.

Skill level	Moderate

Serving size	3
Place of origin	South India, India
Season most suited for consumption	All seasons
Rich in nutrients	Potassium, Calcium, Zinc, Vitamin K

Know your nutrition

Banana: A very good source of potassium, it reduces exercise-related muscle cramps and soreness. It is a nutrient and energy-dense fruit with dietary fiber, so it provides satiety, helps in curing GI disorders, acidity, blood pressure control, and maintains healthy kidney function.

Black sesame seeds: Black sesame seeds are a good source of calcium as they contain heavy amounts of protein, manganese, iron, copper and phosphorous. They are rich in calcium and zinc. They are also a good source of concentrated calories. Black sesame seeds can keep your bones strong and stave off osteoporosis. The sesame seeds also provide the body with vitamin E, which is required for healthy skin. They are also taken as a preferred source of proteins. Black sesame seeds have a strong aroma and good flavour. It is also rich in fatty acids. Black sesame seeds are rich in minerals and preferable dietary fiber.

Cow's ghee: It has a neutral taste. It contains medium and short-chain fatty acids that help to improve digestion, and reduces bowel problems. It also boosts immunity. It contains vitamin K that helps to reduce arthritis and enhances bone health. It also helps in the proper functioning of the heart and boosts good cholesterol levels. It contains omega-6 fatty acid that helps to reduce insulin resistance and lowers blood sugar levels. It also helps in healing external wounds and improves eye health.

Favourable for conditions

GI disorder, Muscle soreness, Osteoporosis, High blood pressure

Calorie count

Serving Size	Energy (Kcal)	Carbohydrate (gm)	Protein (gm)	Fats (gm)
1	206	38	3.1	4
3	618	114.2	9.4	10

Serving Size	Calcium (mg)	Phosphorus (mg)	Total Fiber (mg)	Omega-3 (mg)
1	40.8	21.9	3.8	11.6
3	122.3	65.8	11.5	34.7

Ingredients

Rice flour	1/3 cups
Small bananas (mashed)	2
Black sesame seeds	1 tsp
Cardamom powder	1 tsp
Ginger powder	1 tsp
Cumin powder	1 tsp
Chopped jaggery	1/4 cup
Water	3/4 cup
Ghee	2 tsp

Method

- Take water in a vessel, add jaggery, and heat on medium flame till it turns into a thick syrup.
- Mash bananas in a vessel, add cardamom powder, ginger powder, and cumin powder and mix well.
- Add rice flour to the jaggery syrup. Also add sesame and mix well until it becomes a smooth batter.
- Now, add the banana mixture into the batter and mix well.
- Take an appam pan and it with brush ghee. Pour the batter

into each mould till 3/4 level and cook on a medium flame.
* Turn the appam and cook again till it becomes golden brown. Serve hot.

Healthy cooking tips

* Strain the rice flour to remove any impurities.
* Do not add too much water in the batter. Keep the consistency of the batter smooth.
* Ripe bananas are beneficial for people with diarrhea and raw bananas for constipation.

❧

CARROT AND CORN APPE

Delectable South Indian Appe recipe packed with the goodness of carrot and corn.

Skill level	Easy
Serving size	2
Place of origin	South India
Season most suited for consumption	All seasons
Rich in nutrients	Carbohydrate, calcium, iron, folate, beta carotene, biotin, vitamin K, etc.

Know your nutrition

Black gram (Urad dal): It is a plant-based source of protein, ideal for vegetarians and vegans. It is a source of zinc and potassium. It aids in digestion and prevents anemia. It improves heart health due to the presence of magnesium, fiber and potassium.

Carrot (Gajar): They are a good source of vitamins A and K, biotin, potassium, and vitamin B6. Carrot improves eyesight and immune function, provides satiety and prevents constipation. It also reduces the risk of cancer.

Sweet corn (Bhutta): Sweet corn is a great source of vitamins A and C. They contain a large amount of soluble fiber that helps decrease cholesterol. They increase levels of beneficial antioxidants and phytochemicals. Dietary fiber in the food helps regulate blood sugar levels. Corn is a good source of phenolic flavonoid antioxidant, ferulic acid. The ferulic acid plays a vital role in preventing cancers, aging, and inflammation in humans.

Favourable for conditions

Weight loss, Children, Adolescents, Pregnancy, Bone, Muscle health

Calorie count

Serving Size	Energy (Kcal)	Carbohydrate (gm)	Protein (gm)	Fats (gm)	Calcium (mg)	Sodium (mg)
1	201	35.3	4.7	0.9	25.9	880.1
2	402	70.6	9.5	1.8	51.8	1760.2
Serving Size	Phosphorus (mg)	Total Fiber (mg)	Omega-3 (mg)	Beta-carotene (mcg)	Potassium (mg)	
1	52.9	4.1	50.1	1093.5	266.6	
2	105.9	8.2	100.3	2187	533.2	

Ingredients

Carrot	50 gm
Sweet corn	25 gm
Rice	60 gm
Urad dal	30 gm
Cumin seeds	1-2
Curry leaves	1-2
Hing	A pinch

| Rice bran oil | 1 tsp |
| Salt | ¼ tsp |

Method

- Add raw rice and urad dal in a bowl and soak it for 3-4 hours.
- Drain the water after 3-4 hours and blend them in a blender.
- Keep this mixture aside for 8-9 hours to ferment.
- Boil sweet corn in a pan for 10-15 minutes.
- In a pan add cumin seeds, curry leaves, hing, carrot, and sweet corn.
- Let it cook for 10-15 minutes or until completely cooked with the lid closed.
- Remove from heat and add this mixture to the fermented mixture.
- Heat appe molds that are greased with oil.
- Put the mixture into the molds and let it cook on steam until one side of appe is golden brown.
- Serve hot with chutney.

Healthy cooking tips

- Wash the carrots well and use with skin.
- Do not strain the carrot juice as fiber may be lost.
- Cooking carrots enhance the lycopene content and increase vitamin A availability.

MIX VEGETABLE APPAM

Invigorating Tamil Nadu snacks that is bursting with stimulating vegetables and also nutritiously satisfy cravings.

Skill level	Moderate
Serving size	3
Place of origin	Tamil Nadu, India

Season most suited for consumption	All seasons
Rich in nutrients	Fiber, Vitamin A, C, Iron, Potassium, Magnesium, Protein

Know your nutrition

Cauliflower: Cauliflower is a rich source of flavonoids, which is an antioxidant that helps in reducing free radicals, cancer, heart disease, and neuro-degenerative disease. It also has high amounts of fiber, which provides satiety and decreases digestion related problems.

Broccoli: It helps in reducing cholesterol and lowers blood pressure, reduces the risk of cancer. Broccoli is a good source of several vitamins and minerals such as vitamins A, C and B9, and zinc. It also has a good dose of beta-carotene and lutein that protects the skin and also helps in relieving inflammation.

Bell peppers (Shimla mirch): Bell peppers provide key antioxidants such as lycopene, beta carotene, lutein and zeaxanthin that protects the body from free radicals, helps reduce the risk of cancer, heart disease, and neuro-degenerative disease. It is also rich in vitamin C, vitamin A as well as a moderate source for vitamins E and K, manganese, and potassium. It also has high amounts of fiber that provides fullness to the stomach and decreases digestion-related problems. It protects eyesight and promotes bone health.

Favourable for conditions

Diabetes, Hypertension, Cardiac health, Immunity

Calorie count

Serving Size	Energy (Kcal)	Carbohydrate (gm)	Protein (gm)	Fats (gm)	Calcium (mg)	Phosphorus (mg)
1	219	37.4	8	0.7	36.6	71.9
3	656	112.1	23.9	2.1	109.7	215.7

Serving Size	Iron (mg)	Potassium (mg)	Magnesium (mg)	Total Fiber (mg)	Omega-3 (mg)	Vitamin A (mcg)
1	0.9	313	21	8.7	35.6	114.2
3	2.6	939.1	63.1	26.1	106.9	452.6

Serving Size	Vitamin C (mg)
1	10.4
3	31.2

Ingredients

Cauliflower, raw	1 cup
Broccoli, raw or steamed	¾ cup
Cabbage	½ cup
Capsicum	¼ cup
Semolina	2 tbsp
Carrots, chopped	1/3 cup
Ginger	½ inch
Coriander leaves, chopped	¼ cup
Mint leaves	1 tbsp
Cumin seeds	1/3 tsp
Salt	½ tsp
Amchur powder	1 tsp
Rice flour	2 tbsp
Chickpea flour	2/3 cup
Water	As needed

Method

- Chop the cauliflower, broccoli, cabbage, capsicum and carrot in small pieces and transfer in a bowl. Cut coriander and mint leaves. Add cumin seeds, salt, amchur powder, grated ginger, and semolina. Mix well. Add rice flour, chickpea flour, and water to the bowl and mix it and let the consistency be thick.
- Take appam maker and pour the batter. Let it steam it steam

and cook until it turns golden brown from both sides Serve it with any chutney of your choice.

Healthy cooking tips

- Broccoli is a healthy and versatile vegetable. Wash the vegetable properly. Steam it; do not overcook as it becomes mushy which also has an impact on the nutrients content. Add a pinch of salt while steaming; it brightens the colour.
- Cut the cauliflower and wash carefully to remove worms. Steam it and add a pinch of cinnamon. Do not cover the cabbage initially with a lid while steaming, as it contains sulfur which may cause flatus and bloating.
- Do not sieve the chickpea flour. Let it be a little coarse. Consume it in the afternoon.

❧

RED VELVET APPAM

A vibrant version of South Indian appam, which offers the sweetness of beetroots.

Skill level	Moderate
Serving size	2
Place of origin	Tamil Nadu, India
Season most suited for consumption	All seasons
Rich in nutrients	Potassium, Calcium, Magnesium, Vitamin C, Iron

Know your nutrition

Beetroot: It can lower blood sugar and also improve oxygen use, stamina and exercise performance. It has a high concentration of nitrates. It enhances athletic performance by improving oxygen use and time of exhaustion. It may help fight inflammation and improve digestive health and brain health.

Soya flour: Soybeans are high in protein. Iron and copper help to increase the amount of red blood cells in the body and improves blood circulation. It is rich in folic acid and vitamin B complex that is essential for pregnant women. The impressive levels of zinc, selenium, copper, magnesium, and calcium in soybean help in keeping the bones stronger and healthier. It has a good amount of dietary fiber, which is essential for total body functioning and plays a vital role in the digestive system. It has a good source of MUFA and PUFA, which helps to lower cholesterol in the body. It has high levels of antioxidants that help to kill cancer cells and remove free radicals from the body. It helps to lower blood pressure, has anti-inflammatory effects, reduces risk of osteoporosis, and helps to manage diabetes by increasing insulin receptors.

Favourable for conditions

Women's health, Children, Athletes, Hypertension, Cardiac Health, Tiffin meals

Calorie count

Serving Size	Energy (Kcal)	Carbohydrate (gm)	Protein (gm)	Fats (gm)	Calcium (mg)	Phosphorus (mg)
1	115	10.7	5.2	1.9	29.4	24.3
2	230	21.5	10.4	3.8	58.9	48.7
Serving Size	Iron (mg)	Potassium (mg)	Magnesium (mg)	Total Fiber (mg)	Omega-3 (mg)	Vitamin C (mg)
1	0.5	116.4	8.8	2.3	6.1	0.2
2	1.1	232.8	17.6	4.7	12.2	0.5
Serving Size	Folate (mg)					
1	15.4					
2	30.9					

Ingredients

Beetroot (boiled and grated)	50 gm
Rice flour	10 gm
Urad dal (split black lentil) flour	15 gm
Soya flour	15 gm
Sesame seeds (til)	1 ½ tsp
Oil	1 tsp
Salt	½ tsp

Method

- Combine urad dal flour, soya flour, rice flour, beetroot (boiled and grated), and sesame seeds with 1 ¼ cup of water in a deep bowl and make a pouring consistency batter.
- Grease mini appam pan with ½ tsp oil and pour the batter in each mold.
- Cook until they become golden brown in colour from both sides and serve with chutney of your choice.

Healthy cooking tips

- Wash beetroot properly, pressure cook and then remove the peel.
- Consume urad dal only in the afternoon.
- You can boil the sesame and then make a paste to make this recipe.

❦

VEGETABLE APPAM

Delectable authentic South Indian recipe that has a blend of stimulating vegetables—an ideal nutritive snack.

Skill level	Easy
Serving size	4
Place of origin	South India, India

Season most suited for consumption	All seasons
Rich in nutrients	Iron, Magnesium, Phosphorus, Folate, Zinc, Vitamin C, Beta-carotene

Know your nutrition

Sodium chloride: Sodium is an electrolyte that facilitates nerve impulses and regulates body functions such as heart rate, digestion, respiration, brain activity, and blood pressure. It helps to maintain the fluid balance in the body.

Sesame oil: It contains sesamol and sesaminol, two antioxidants that help to reduce cell damage by free radicals and protect against oxidative damage. It helps to reduce inflammation and prevents arthritis. It is rich in omega-6 fatty acids that help to prevent heart disease, cancer and reduces cholesterol and regulates blood sugar levels. It contains collagen that helps to heal wounds and burns. It also improves hair quality and provides relief from other joint pains.

Favourable for conditions

Digestion, Diabetes, Hypertension, Cardiac health, Tiffin snack

Calorie count

Serving Size	Energy (Kcal)	Carbohydrate (gm)	Protein (gm)	Fats (gm)	Calcium (mg)	Phosphorus (mg)	Iron (mg)
1	239	33.9	6.3	1.8	14.2	56.5	0.6
4	955.2	135.8	25.4	7.2	56.9	226.1	2.4

Serving Size	Potassium (mg)	Magnesium (mg)	Total Fiber (mg)	Omega-3 (mg)	Beta-carotene (mcg)	Vitamin C (mg)	Folate (mg)
1	250	12	4	18	546.6	3.9	13.4
4	1000.6	48.1	16.1	72	2186.5	15.8	53.7

Ingredients

Idli batter	3 cups
Tomato	1
Carrot	¼ cup
Capsicum	1 (1/4 cup)
Salt	¼ tsp
Green coriander	2 tbsp
Sesame Oil	2 tbsp

Method

- Mix finely chopped tomatoes, capsicum, salt, and green coriander in the idli batter.
- Preheat appam maker and grease the mold with oil.
- Take idli batter mixture in a spoon and pour in the molds.
- Cover and cook for 2 minutes on low flame.
- When the appam turns golden brown from beneath flip the sides.
- Cover again to cook for 2 more minutes.
- Cook until appam turns golden brown on both sides.
- Serve with any chutney of your choice.

Healthy cooking tips

- Soak the urad dal well; at least 6 to 8 hours of soaking is required.
- Consume the urad dal only in the afternoon.
- Soak it overnight and discard the water because the water above will have a white frothy layer that creates flatulence. Wash well and cook it.
- Urad dal can be used as part of the tempering in a lot of dals and chutneys because it gives a nice crunch and increases the protein content.
- Cooking carrots enhances the lycopene content and increases vitamin A availability.

• Always measure salt using level spoons. Do not heap spoons.

9. DHOKLA

GRAIN DHOKLA

A nourishing version of Gujarati dhokla that is a simple, quick and blend of highly nutritive lentils.

Skill level	Moderate
Serving size	4
Place of origin	Gujarat, India
Season most suited for consumption	All seasons
Rich in nutrients	Calcium, Iron, Potassium, Magnesium, Fiber

Know your nutrition

Split Red gram (Masoor dal): It is a plant-based source of protein, ideal for vegetarians and vegans. It aids in digestion. It is a good source of zinc and vitamin B1. It helps maintain cholesterol levels. It also has anti-ageing properties.

Rice bran oil (Chawal ki bhusi ka tel): It has a neutral taste. It contains oryzanol, the antioxidant that helps to lower cholesterol. It contains vitamin E that helps to boost immunity and helps to reduce weight and aids in good immune function. It has tocotrienols, oryzanol, and plant sterols. It also helps to reduce insulin resistance and lowers blood sugar levels. It has anti-inflammatory properties that help to reduce heart disease and cancer.

Asafoetida (Hing): The Charak Samhita mentions it for treatment of respiratory, stomach and children's disorders, impotency, women's ailments, toothache and cholera. Its resinous gum is said to help patients with anemia, intestinal worms, aches and pains and fevers.

Favourable for conditions

Diabetes, Hypertension, Cardiac health, Weight loss

Calorie count

Serving Size	Energy (Kcal)	Carbohydrate (gm)	Protein (gm)	Fats (gm)	Calcium (mg)	Phosphorus (mg)
1	187	20.6	0.7	4.4	64.6	80.2
4	749	82.5	3	17.6	258.4	320.8

Serving Size	Iron (mg)	Potassium (mg)	Magnesium (mg)	Total Fiber (mg)	Omega-3 (mg)	Vitamin A (mcg)
1	1.6	356.6	26.9	6.1	392.7	66.9
4	6.3	1426.6	107.7	24.4	1571	267.8

Serving Size	Folate (mg)
	26.3
	105.4

Ingredients

For dhokla:

Split Bengal gram (chana dal)	25 gm
Black gram lentil (urad dal)	25 gm
Split red lentil (masoor dal)	25 gm
Yellow lentil (Mung dal)	25 gms
Split green Mung dal (chilte dal)	50 gm
Spinach, one big bunch	50 gm
Salt	½ tsp

For garnishing:

Rice Bran Oil	2 tsp
Mustard seeds	1 tsp
Cumin seeds	1 tsp
Black sesame seeds	1 tbsp
Flaxseeds	1 tbsp

Coriander leaves	2 tbsp
Asafoetida	A pinch
Coconut flakes	2 tbsp

Method

- Soak all five dals for about 4-5 hrs. Then drain the water and grind all the soaked dals with salt.
- Wash the spinach and grind to a purée.
- Add spinach purée in a dal mixture and make a batter of a medium consistency.
- Grease the base as well as sides of the pan before steaming the dhokla.
- Take a pressure cooker and add 2.5 cups of water and place the stand inside it. Put the pot on medium flame and let the water come to a boil.
- Pour the batter in the greased pan and let it steam for 7-8 minutes.
- Once done, use a knife to cut the dhokla into medium pieces.
- For tempering, heat 1 tbsp oil in a tadka pan.
- Add mustard seeds, flaxseeds, cumin seeds, black sesame seeds, curry leaves and add a pinch of asafoetida.
- Fry a few seconds till the curry leaves become crispy.
- And the tadka evenly on the dhokla, garnish with chopped coconut and coriander leaves and serve it.

Healthy cooking tips

- Wash well and discard the water. Discarding water may reduce bloating and can also reduce uric acid levels.
- Eat dals only in the afternoon, as at night they may cause bloating and flatulence.
- It should be eaten as it is or it can be powdered and added to dals and vegetables.

MIX VEGETABLE DHOKLA

A steamed, fluffy Gujarati delicacy that is teeming with fiber, protein, all beneficial nutrients and superfoods.

Skill level	Moderate
Serving size	6
Place of origin	Gujarat, India
Season most suited for consumption	All seasons
Rich in nutrients	Protein and vitamin A

Know your nutrition

Rice: White rice is a good source of magnesium, phosphorus, manganese, selenium, iron, folic acid, thiamine and niacin, and additionally, its low fiber content may help with digestive issues.

Black gram (Urad dal): It is a plant-based source of protein, ideal for vegetarians and vegans. It is a source of zinc and potassium. It aids in digestion and prevents anemia. It improves heart health due to the presence of magnesium, fiber and potassium.

Carrot (Gajar): They are a good source of vitamin A, biotin, vitamin K, potassium, and vitamin B6. Improves eyesight and immune function and provides satiety and prevents constipation. It also reduces the risk of cancer.

Favourable for conditions

Eye disease, Constipation, Heart health

Calorie count

Serving Size	Energy (Kcal)	Carbohy-drate (gm)	Protein (gm)	Fats (gm)	Calcium (mg)	Phosphorus (mg)	Total Fiber (mg)	Omega-3 (mg)	Vitamin A (mcg)
1	190	37.1	5.6	0.1	13.4	66.3	4.1	61.8	82.2
6	1141	222.6	33.4	0.8	80.4	397.7	24.7	371.1	493.4

Ingredients

Rice	2 cups
Urad dal	120 g
Carrot	50 g
Peas	25 g
French beans	50 g
Salt	½ tsp

For tempering:

Oil	½ tsp
Mustard seeds	¼ tsp
Curry leaves	4-5

Method

- Soak the rice and urad dal for 6-8 hours. Add salt and grind to a paste.
- Chop the vegetables into small pieces and mix them in the batter.
- Take a plate with raised edges and put the batter in.
- Steam the dhoklas.
- For tempering, place a small kadhai, add oil and mustard seeds and wait till they pop.
- Then, turn off the flame and add the curry leaves.
- Spread the tempered mixture over the warm dhoklas and serve hot.

Healthy cooking tips

- Use parboiled rice instead of basmati rice. Do not strain the rice water away. Use it in other preparations like soups.
- Soak the urad dal well for at least 6 to 8 hrs.
- Wash the carrots well and use them without the skin.
- Always measure salt using level spoons and do not heap spoons.
- Homemakers can use small spoons for measuring to consciously reduce the quantity of salt consumed daily

10. IDLI

KANCHIPURAM IDLI

Scrumptious South Indian idlis

Skill level	Moderate
Serving size	4
Place of origin	Tamil Nadu, India
Season most suited for consumption	All seasons
Rich in nutrients	Fiber, Beta Carotene, Vitamin B9, Potassium

Know your Nutrition:

White rice: White rice is a good source of magnesium, phosphorus, manganese, selenium, iron, folic acid, thiamine, and niacin, and additionally, its low fiber content may help with digestive issues.

Urad dal: Urad dal is a plant-based source of protein, ideal for vegetarians and vegans. It is a source of zinc and potassium. It aids in digestion and prevents anemia. It improves heart health due to the presence of magnesium, fiber, and potassium.

Cashew nuts: Cashew nut contains copper and iron that support healthy blood formation. It helps to reduce blood pressure and cholesterol levels as it contains potassium, vitamin E, B6. It contains lutein and zeaxanthin, which act as antioxidants and are good for the eyes.

Favourable for conditions

Gluten free, children, Senior citizens, Pregnancy, Lactation, Digestion, Athletes, Anemia

Calorie count

Serving Size	Energy (Kcal)	Carbohydrate (gm)	Protein (gm)	Fats (gm)	Calcium (mg)
1	212	20.7	4.4	11.2	14.7
4	848	83.12	17.5	44.9	59

Serving Size	Phosphorus (mg)	Total Fiber (mg)	Omega-3 (mg)	Potassium (mg)	Beta-carotene (mcg)
1	45.8	2.7	45.9	184.9	48.6
4	180.3	11	183.6	739.8	194.6

Serving Size	Folate (mcg)
	9.4
	37.7

Ingredients:

Urad dal	1 cup
Rice	1 cup
Chana dal	1 tsp
Curd	¾ cup
Cashewnuts	5
Coconut freshly grated	½
Black pepper	½ tsp
Curry leaves	3 to 4
Salt	1 tsp
Ghee	2 tbsp
Oil	For greasing

Method:

- Wash and soak the urad dal and rice together and chana dal separately for at least 4 hours.
- Grind the urad dal and rice to a coarse paste. Leave it at least for 6 hours.
- Add the curd, cashew nuts, coconut, pepper powder, curry

leaves, ghee, salt, and the soaked chana dal and mix well.

- Pour a little batter into greased idli molds and steam for 10 to 12 minutes.
- Repeat with the remaining batter to make more idlis. Serve hot with a chutney of your choice.

Healthy cooking tips:

- Soak the dals well for at least 6-8 hrs.
- Soak overnight and discard the water. Wash well and cook it.
- Urad dal can be used as a part of tempering in a lot of dals and chutneys because it gives a nice crunch and increases the protein content. Grill, boil, steam and bake instead of frying where possible.

PANIYARAM

Lip-smacking South Indian snack recipe that stimulates the taste buds.

Skill level	Easy
Serving size	2
Place of origin	South India, India
Season most suited for consumption	All seasons
Rich in nutrients	Magnesium, Phosphorus, Protein, Zinc, Potassium, Arginine

Know your nutrition

White rice: White rice is a good source of magnesium, phosphorus, manganese, selenium, iron, folic acid, thiamine, and niacin, and additionally, its fiber content may help with digestive issues.

Black gram (Urad dal): It is a plant-based source of protein, ideal for vegetarians and vegans. It is a source of Zinc and Potassium. It aids in digestion and prevents anemia. It improves heart health due to the presence of magnesium, fiber and potassium.

Coconut: Coconut is low in carbohydrates and high in fiber, which helps stabilize blood sugar. Coconut has an antidiabetic effect due to its arginine content. It is high in antioxidants, which also prevent oxidative damage. It has a beneficial effect on heart health and is also good for skin and hair health.

Favourable for conditions

Anemia, Digestive issues, Heart disease, Diabetes

Calorie count

Serving Size	Energy (Kcal)	Carbohydrate (gm)	Protein (gm)	Fats (gm)	Calcium (mg)	Phosphorus (mg)	Total Fiber (mg)	Omega-3 (mg)
1	313	48.3	6.4	8.6	17.3	71.8	5.3	50
2	625	96.6	12.7	17.3	34.6	143.6	10.7	100

Ingredients

Rice	2 cup
Urad dal	2 tbsp
Grated coconut	½ cup
Ginger (grated)	½ inch
Chopped curry leaves	2 tsp
Salt	1 tsp

Method

- In a blender, make the idli batter using overnight soaked rice and urad dal. Add all the remaining ingredients in the batter and mix well.
- Heat the Paniyaram pan, grease it, pour the batter into the pan and cook. Cover it with a lid and cook for 3 mins.

- Remove the lid, turn the Paniyaram and cook till it turns brown.
- Serve them with coconut chutney or sambar.

Healthy cooking tips

- Cover it and cook, so that the Paniyaram gets cooked completely well from inside.
- Use parboiled rice instead of Basmati rice.
- Soak the dal well for atleast for 6-8 hrs.
- Soak overnight and discard the water.
- Many people discard the curry leaf from dals and vegetables. Dry roast on a tawa, powder the curry leaves and add in the recipe.
- Coconut itself contains a good amount of oil so while using coconut, use less oil.

SANWA IDLI

An appetizing steamed fluffy idli recipe that is prepared with richness of barnyard millet.

Skill level High

Serving size	2
Place of origin	South India, India
Season most suited for consumption	All seasons
Rich in nutrients	Vitamin A, Phosphorus, And Omega 3

Know your nutrition

Barnyard millet: It is a rich source of fiber, which helps in facilitating your digestion, managing obesity and regulating blood sugar levels. It is a rich source of protein, which helps in building muscles, cell regeneration and gives you a feeling of satiety. It is packed with various minerals and vitamins, which help in keeping the body healthy.

Urad dal: It is a plant-based source of protein, ideal for vegetarians and vegans. It is a source of zinc and potassium. It aids in digestion and prevents anemia. It improves heart health due to the presence of magnesium, fiber and potassium.

Favourable for conditions

Gluten free, Weight loss, Diabetes, Anemia, Cardiac health, Women's health, PCOS, Pregnancy, Lactation

Calorie count

Serving Size	Energy (Kcal)	Carbohydrate (gm)	Protein (gm)	Fats (gm)	Calcium (mg)
1	149	29.8	6.3	1.4	25.2
2	372	59.6	12.7	2.9	50.4
Serving Size	Phosphorus (mg)	Total Fiber (mg)	Omega-3 (mg)	Beta-carotene (mcg)	
1	80.6	4.3	43.3	51.6	
2	161.3	8.6	86.6	103.1	

Ingredients

Urad dal	½ cup
Sanwa (Barnyard millet)	½ cup
Water	4 cup
Oil	1 tsp
Mustard Seeds	½ tsp
Sesame seeds	½ tsp
Fresh coriander leaves	For garnishing
Salt	¼ tsp

Method

- Wash and soak urad dal overnight.

- Wash and soak sanwa overnight.
- In a mixer grind the dal, using some of the water, as and when required.
- Separately grind sanwa in the same way.
- Mix dal and sanwa batter together and keep it aside, covered, to rise.
- Keep the batter in a warm place for another 8 hours approximately.
- Mix the batter with turmeric and salt.
- Take an idli stand and apply some oil at the bottom. Pour the batter and steam the idlis.
- Carefully remove from container.
- Serve them with sambhar and chutney.
- Another option is to cut the idlis in four pieces.
- In a kadhai, add oil and heat it to make a baghar with curry leaves, mustard seeds, jeera, black and white sesame seeds.
- Add cut idlis in the kadhai and stir till the idlis are coated with seeds.
- Garnish with green coriander leaves.
- Serve hot with mint chutney.

Healthy cooking tips

- Sanwa puffs can be used in replacement to kurmura.
- Good gluten-free replacement to the calorie-dense refined flour.
- It can be replaced by jowar and ragi.
- It can be sprouted before using it.

11. MUTHIYA

DUDHI MULTIGRAIN MUTHIYA

Tempting muthiya is a Gujarati staple recipe teeming with fiber from grains and leafy greens.

Skill level	Moderate
Serving size	2
Place of origin	Gujarat, India
Season most suited for consumption	All seasons
Rich in nutrients	Fiber, Iron, Vitamin C

Know your nutrition

Wheat: Whole wheat is important because it is high in fiber, vitamins, antioxidants and minerals. It lowers the risk of diabetes, heart disease and high blood pressure. It is known for controlling obesity.

Jowar: It is a rich source of fiber, which helps in facilitating the digestion, managing obesity and regulating blood sugar levels. Jowar is also a rich source of protein that helps in muscle building, cell regeneration and gives a feeling of satiety. Jowar is packed with various minerals and vitamins, which help in keeping the body healthy.

Bottle gourd (Lauki): Bottle gourd is a modest source of vitamin C, which is one of the most powerful antioxidants. It helps the body to fight against the free radicals, cancer and inflammation. It is even a good source of calcium and has a high content of water. It is rich in dietary fiber that helps in curing indigestion and constipation.

Favourable for conditions

Diabetes, Poor gut health, Obesity, Cancer

Calorie count

Serving Size	Energy (Kcal)	Carbohydrate (gm)	Protein (gm)	Fats (gm)	Iron (mg)
1	435	72.4	8.5	8.3	2.6
2	870	144.8	16.9	16.9	5.2

Serving Size	Calcium (mg)	Phosphorus (mg)	Total Fiber (mg)	Omega-3 (mg)
1	63.6	178.3	9.9	108.5
2	127.1	356.7	19.8	216.9

Ingredients

Wheat flour, jowar flour	200 gm, each
Dudhi	250 gm
Turmeric	1 tsp
Salt	¼ tsp
Jeera powder	1 tsp
Sugar	1 tsp
Coriander	Few
Lemon	½
Ginger	1 cm
Sesame seeds	2 tsp
Cumin seeds	1 tsp
Mustard seeds	1 tsp
Curry leaves	1-2
Oil	1 tbsp
Water	

Method

- Sieve all the flours in the bowl, then grate dudhi into it.
- Add all the masalas—salt, turmeric, jeera powder, sugar, lemon, coriander, and some oil and knead the dough.
- Add water when required; dough should be hard.
- Divide the dough into equal portions and roll them into long strands.
- In a vessel add some water and preheat it, then put the rolls to steam and cover for 15-20 minutes.
- Once they are steamed well, cut into small pieces, dividing in equal proportions.
- In a small dekchi, heat the oil, add cumin seeds, mustard seeds

allow them to crackle for a minute and then add curry leaves and sesame seeds, then add all the pieces and mix well. Serve hot.

Healthy cooking tips

- Bottle gourd is used for making salads and juices. It is a healthy vegetable widely used for weight loss. It is low in calories and can be cooked in minimal oil. The peels can be used to make chutney, causing zero waste.

- Jowar puffs can be used in replacement for kurmura and it is a good gluten-free replacement to the calorie-dense refined flour. It is very versatile and can be used in roti, bhakri, muthiya, etc. and ideal for Irritable Bowel Syndrome (IBS). Atta can be used in porridges, thepla and muthiya.

METHI MUTHIYA

Wholesome Gujarati muthiya enriched with organic flavour from methi leaves and indigenous spices.

Skill level	Moderate
Serving size	4
Place of origin	Gujarat, India
Season most suited for consumption	All seasons
Rich in nutrients	Magnesium, Potassium, Protein, Vitamin C, Calcium

Know your nutrition

Fenugreek leaves (Methi): It lowers blood glucose levels and blood lipids as it is rich in magnesium and antioxidants. It also acts as antioxidant and is rich in fiber that gives satiety. It is the best source of iron, hence recommended to anemic patients. It is also antibacterial and antifungal.

Dates (Khajur): Dates contain polyphenols that protect against Alzheimer's disease and colon cancer. High content of iron in dates prevents anemia. Dates have a low glycemic, index which controls blood sugar level. High content of fiber in dates prevent constipation. Calcium and phosphorus in dates promote bone health. It may also promote brain health. Date contains potassium, which lowers bold pressure.

Lemon (Nimbu): Lemon has vitamin C. Sprinkling some over iron-rich foods would aid in better absorption of iron from the source. It has anti-viral and anti-inflammatory properties and it helps in boosting immunity, and lowers the risk of heart diseases like atherosclerosis, diabetes, cancers and kidney stones.

Favourable for conditions

Diabetes, Bone disorders, Anemia, Infection, Cancer, Heart disease

Calorie count

Serving Size	Energy (Kcal)	Carbohydrate (gm)	Protein (gm)	Fats (gm)	Calcium (mg)	Phosphorus (mg)	Folate (mcg)
1	208	28.8	7.1	5	38.5	58.4	116.4
4	834	115.1	28.5	20.2	154.2	233.8	465.7

Serving Size	Potassium (mg)	Sodium (mg)	Magnesium (mg)	Total Fiber (mg)	Omega-3 (mg)	Vitamin A (mcg)	
1	98.2	439.2	41.2	5.7	8.6	53.4	
4	392.8	1757	164.7	22.8	34.6	213.7	

Ingredients

Chickpea flour	1 cup
Fenugreek leaves, finely chopped	½ cup
Lemon juice	¾ tsp
Dates powder	1 tbsp
Ginger paste	½ tsp

Turmeric powder	¼ tsp
Sesame seeds	2 tsp
Ghee	1 tbsp
Salt	½ tsp

Method

- In a bowl, take chickpea flour, fenugreek leaves, dates powder, ginger, turmeric powder and salt. Mix well using a few drops of water only if needed, then shape it into small balls and steam in a steamer.
- Put a fork in it and check, if it comes out dry the it is done.
- In a pan, put ghee, add sesame seeds and fry till brown. Spread on the muthiya and serve.

Healthy cooking tips

- Fenugreek works as a flavouring agent, in both fresh and dried forms. Fresh methi leaves can be used as a vegetable, with potatoes, or with besan; and in dals, rotis, theplas, and muthiyas. Dry kasuri methi can be added to dals and curries to give a distinct aroma and increase iron levels in one's body.
- Flours should not be made and stored for a long time in the fridge as their nutritional value decreases. Don't use finely sieved flour.
- Dates have a low glycemic index and are high in fiber.
- Avoid consumption of ghee in large quantities as it may elevate cholesterol.

❦

RASA WALA MUTHIYA

An appetizing traditional Gujarati recipe, which is transformed by using brown rice.

Skill level   Moderate

Serving size	2
Place of origin	Gujarat, India
Season most suited for consumption	All seasons
Rich in nutrients	Fiber, Prebiotics, Protein

Know your nutrition

Brown rice: Brown rice is a wholegrain and a good source of magnesium, phosphorus, selenium, thiamine, niacin, vitamin B6, and manganese, and the fiber in it helps manage cholesterol, moves waste through the digestive tract, give satiety, and helps to prevent the formation of blood clots.

Favourable for conditions

Diabetes, Constipation, Obesity

Calorie count

Serving Size	Energy (Kcal)	Carbohydrate (gm)	Protein (gm)	Fats (gm)	Calcium (mg)	Phosphorus (mg)	Total Fiber (mg)	Omega 3 (mg)
1	231	30.7	5.6	8.4	93.8	14.5	1.8	82.4
2	462	61.3	11.3	16.5	187.6	28.9	3.1	6789.8

Ingredients

Brown Rice	60 gm
Wheat flour	15 gm
Buttermilk	500 ml
Coriander	a few
Salt	¼ tsp
Turmeric	2 tsp
Dhana jeera	2 tsp
Mustard seeds	1 tsp
Cumin seeds	1 tsp
Filtered oil	1 tbsp

Method

- Wash the brown rice and boil it.
- Spread the brown rice on the dish and leave it to cool.
- Once it is cool, add salt, turmeric, jeera powder, wheat flour and mix it well.
- Divide the mixture in equal portions and give them a round or oval shape.
- In a dekchi, heat the oil. Add cumin seeds and mustard seeds, allow them to crackle. Once they start crackling, add buttermilk and stir well. Add turmeric, salt, jeera powder and coriander.
- Allow the muthiya to cook for some time and then serve hot.

Healthy cooking tips

- Do not sieve wheat atta; retain the bran.
- Use Punjabi atta or Jada atta.
- While sieving, remove stones and impurities but retain fiber.
- Do not use refined flour.
- Add other grain flours to make it a multigrain atta which is far superior in nutrition.

C. INTERNATIONAL BREAKFAST/EXERCISE MEALS

APPLE CHIA AND FLAXSEEDS OATMEAL

Easy wholesome breakfast, rich in fiber, omega 3, vitamins and essential nutrients.

Skill level	Easy
Serving size	2
Place of origin	Eastern Europe
Season most suited for consumption	All seasons
Rich in nutrients	Fiber, Omega 3, Beta carotene

Know your nutrition

Walnuts contain bioactive compounds that have anti-cancer properties. They also contain a good amount of omega-3 fatty acids which improve brain functions and may help alleviate depression and age-related decline in brain functions. Omega-3 fatty acids, also help reduce inflammation. They also promote a healthy gut.

Favourable for conditions

Athletes, Children, Adolescents, Pregnancy, Bone, and Muscle health

Calorie count

Serving size	Energy (kcal)	Carbohydrates (gm)	Protein (gm)	Fats (gm)	Calcium (gm)
1	275	28.1	8	12.9	145.1
2	551	56.2	16.1	25.9	290.2
Phosphorus (gm)	Iron (gm)	Fiber (gm)	Omega-3 (mg)	Beta carotene (mcg)	
140.5	1.2	5.2	1789.8	12.3	
281.1	2.5	10.4	3579.6	24.7	

Ingredients

Oats	1/3 cup
Milk	1 cup
Apple	½ cup
Chia seeds	½ tbsp
Flaxseeds	1 tbsp
Walnuts	2 pcs
Honey	1 tsp

Method

• Cook milk and oats for 5-7 minutes with chia seeds.

- Add flaxseeds, apple, walnuts, and honey.
- Serve immediately.

Healthy cooking tips

- Use steel-cut rolled oats and not processed oats or instant oats.
- Soak oats in water for 10 minutes and then use them in preparations. E.g.: Porridge
- If used as a powder in a soup or vegetable, the oats should be nicely dry roasted before powdering, which can then be added to the preparation as a thickening agent.

MANGO AND OAT PARFAIT

Appealing parfait with the goodness of seasonal fruitiness from mangoes and fiber-rich oats.

Skill level	Easy
Serving size	1
Place of origin	France
Season most suited for consumption	All seasons
Rich in nutrients	Magnesium

Know your nutrition

Mango is a low-calorie fruit that is high in fiber, so it improves digestive health. It is a great source of vitamins C and A and hence it can boost immune health and prevent damage from muscular degeneration and cancer. It also contains folate, B6, iron, and a little calcium, zinc, and vitamin E. It is a good source of energy and it can also promote healthy skin and hair.

Favourable for conditions

Athletes, Children, Adolescents, Pregnancy, Bone, and Muscle health

Calorie count

Serving size	Energy (kcal)	Carbohydrates (gm)	Protein (gm)	Fats (gm)	Calcium (gm)
1	218	26	6.4	8.5	160.2
Serving size	Iron (gm)	Phosphorus (gm)	Omega-3 (mg)	Magnesium (mg)	Fiber (gm)
1	1.9	152.4	15.2	31.5	8.6

Ingredients

Oats	20 gm
Curd	30 gm
Mango	25 gm
Chia/Sabja seeds	2 tbsp

Method

- Take a glass jar or a bowl.
- Add curd to it. Mix the oats.
- In the next layer, add soaked chia seeds.
- Top it with dry fruits.
- Refrigerate it the night before.
- Garnish with mango just before serving.

Healthy cooking tips

- Aamras can be prepared or eaten as a whole fruit or can be added into smoothies, shrikhands, ice-creams or yogurt.
- Diabetes patient should avoid consuming more than half or 1 mango at a time.
- Avoid eating mangoes and aamras during mealtime because it can increase sugar levels.

- It is good to consume it as a pre-workout meal.

✿

MUESLI CHIA SEED AND DRY FRUIT JAR

A vivacious jar recipe blended with a fruity flavour, fiber-rich muesli, and the sweetness from honey.

Skill level	Easy
Serving size	3
Place of Origin	Germany
Season Most Suited for Consumption	Summer
Rich in Nutrients	Vitamins, Omega 3 Fatty Acid, Calcium, Phosphorus

Know your nutrition

Banana: A very good source of potassium, hence reduces exercise-related muscle cramps and soreness. It is a nutrient- and energy-dense fruit with dietary fiber so it provides satiety, helps cure GI, acidity, blood pressure control, and maintains healthy kidney function.

Cranberry: Cranberries are rich in ascorbic acid, fat-soluble vitamin E, manganese and have polyphenols such as quercetin and myricetin that collectively have anti-inflammatory, anti-atherogenic properties and are known to reduce postprandial blood glucose. As a good source of fiber, they help to relieve constipation. They also reduce the adherence of E. coli bacteria in the gut particularly due to the presence of a particular polyphenol and A-type proanthocyanins.

Chia seeds: Chia seeds have a high amount of antioxidants that have anti-aging properties. Chia seeds are also an excellent source of plant protein that may help in muscle recovery. High fiber and protein content in chia seeds may help to lose weight. They have a high amount of Omega-3 fatty acids that reduce inflammation. Calcium, phosphorus and magnesium content in chia seeds promote bone health.

Favourable for conditions

Athletes, Children, Adolescents, Working executives

Calorie count

Serving Size	Energy (Kcal)	Carbohydrate (gm)	Protein (gm)	Fats (gm)	Calcium (mg)
1	263	45.7	6.4	7.5	113.8
3	789	137	19.1	22.4	341.5
Serving Size	Phosphorus (mg)	Total Fiber (mg)	Omega-3 (mg)	Folic acid (mcg)	Magnesium (mg)
1	143.5	6.6	14	236.3	36.9
3	430.6	19.8	42	708.9	110.8

Ingredients

Muesli	100 gm
Chia Seeds, soaked in ½ cup water	50 grm
Curd	½ cup
Cinnamon powder	1 tsp
Ripe banana, sliced	2
Honey	1 tbsp
Salt	¼ tsp
Prunes, chopped	1 tbsp
Cranberries	1 tbsp
Pomegranate seed powder	1 tsp

Method

• Soak the chia seeds in water for 10 minutes and then mix with yogurt, honey and cinnamon powder. Keep it in the refrigerator to set.

- Take a jar, add a tablespoon of chia seeds mixed with yogurt, and then add in the muesli and finally some chopped banana, prunes, cranberries and pomegranate seed powder. Repeat the process until the jar is full.

Healthy cooking tips

- Make sure you use fresh fruits.
- Sabja seeds can be used instead of chia seeds, as they are a good source of minerals, calcium and magnesium that are essential for our bone health and muscle function, while the iron is vital for red blood cell production. They are also high in fiber.
- Kiwis can be used as an alternative fruit as they are an excellent source of vitamins. They prevent bleeding gums and are rich in potassium. Their seeds contain abundant amounts of vitamin E.

D. INTERNATIONAL SNACKS

1. MISCELLANEOUS

CHEESE CORN SPINACH PATTY

Delectable snack prepared with vibrant ingredient such as spinach, mint and corn kernels.

Skill level	Easy
Serving size	4
Place of origin	Mexico
Season most suited for consumption	All seasons
Rich in nutrients	Vitamin A, C, Potassium, Manganese, Fiber

Know your nutrition

Sweet potato (Shakarkand): It's rich in fiber, a good source of vitamins A, C and B6, potassium, copper, and manganese. It also promotes gut health. It is said to have cancer-fighting properties and enhances brain function. It also supports the immune system.

Sweet corn (Bhutta): Sweet corn is a great source of vitamins C and A. They also contain large amounts of soluble fiber, help decrease cholesterol, and increase levels of beneficial antioxidants and phytochemicals. Dietary fiber in the food helps regulate blood sugar levels. Corn is a good source of the phenolic flavonoid antioxidant, ferulic acid, which plays a vital role in preventing cancers, aging, and inflammation in humans.

Cow milk paneer: Ideal source of protein for vegetarians, which is easily absorbed in the body. It is rich in calcium and vitamin D. It improves digestion and helps in weight loss. Also helps in preventing pernicious anemia.

Favourable for conditions

Hypertension, Cardiac health, Anemia, Children

Calorie count

Serving Size	Energy (Kcal)	Carbohydrate (gm)	Protein (gm)	Fats (gm)	Calcium (mg)	Phosphorus (mg)
1	99	10.1	3.4	1.5	44	44.1
4	398	40.5	13.5	6.1	176.3	176.4

Serving Size	Total Fiber (mg)	Omega-3 (mg)	Potassium (mg)	Magnesium (mg)	Vitamin A (mcg)	Vitamin C (mg)
1	2.5	47.1	293.8	17	407.5	4.1
4	9.9	188.4	1175.2	68.2	1630	16.5

Ingredients

Sweet potato	100 gm
Boiled sweet corn kernels	50 gm
Spinach, chopped	100 gm
Spring onion leaves, chopped	20 gm
Fresh mint leaves, chopped	10 gm
Fresh coriander leaves, chopped	20 gm
Amchur powder	1 tsp
Salt	½ tsp
Paneer, grated	100 gm
Oil	1 tbsp

Method

- Chop spinach, spring onion leaves, mint leaves, coriander leaves and transfer in a bowl.
- Pressure cook sweet corn and sweet potato, smash the sweet potato and add both in a bowl.
- Add salt, amchur powder and grated paneer to the bowl and mix all the ingredients properly. Now give it a patty shape.
- Take the pan and put a little oil in it. Shallow fry the patties from both sides until golden brown and serve with any chutney of your choice.

Healthy cooking tips

- Sweet potato is very high in fiber and a good replacement for potatoes. It can also be used as a thickener. Do not roast sweet potato as it increases the dietary AGE; instead, steam before cooking. Use fresh coriander leaves and wash and clean them properly.
- Sweet corn husk is to be removed properly. Remove the silky threads and then pressure-cook it.
- When making paneer at home, try to use cow's milk because paneer made from cow's milk is lower in fat compared to that

made of cow milk. Use this homemade paneer in various forms like cubed, crumbled or grated, to make parathas and mithai. If you are vegan, you can use soya milk or almond milk paneer.

❧

IDLI BURGER

An Indian version of the no-bread burger. Appealing vegetarian patty sandwiched between two idlis.

Skill level	Moderate
Serving size	4
Place of origin	Germany and the US
Season most suited for consumption	All seasons
Rich in nutrients	Protein, Dietary Fiber, Vitamins C and B-Complex Vitamins, Sodium, Potassium, Beta Carotene, Antioxidants

Know your nutrition

White rice: White rice is a good source of magnesium, phosphorus, manganese, selenium, iron, folic acid, thiamine and niacin and additionally, its low fiber content may help with digestive issues.

Black gram (Urad dal): It is a plant-based source of protein, ideal for vegetarians and vegans. It is a source of zinc and potassium. It aids in digestion and prevents anemia. It improves heart health due to the presence of magnesium, fiber and potassium.

Lettuce: It acts as anti-inflammatory agent that reduces inflammation. It induces sleep as it contains lactucarium that acts on the central nervous system to produce pain-relieving and sedative effects. It controls anxiety due to its sedative and anxiolytic properties. It also prevents cancer as it inhibits the growth of leukemia cells and breast cancer cells.

Favourable for conditions

Weight loss, Diabetes, Children, Adolescents, Gluten free, Athletes

Calorie count

Serving Size	Energy (Kcal)	Carbohydrate (gm)	Protein (gm)	Fats (gm)	Calcium (mg)	Phosphorus (mg)
1	313	57.2	8	2.9	53.2	108.8
4	1252	229.1	32	11.9	213.1	435.5

Serving Size	Total Fiber (mg)	Omega-3 (mg)	Sodium (mg)	Potassium (mg)	Beta carotene (mcg)	Vitamin C (mg)
1	4.3	26.6	554.5	420.6	514.8	3.3
4	17.4	106.6	2218	1682.4	2059.3	13.4

Ingredients

For idli:

Unpolished rice	1 cup
Raddle	¼ cup
Yoghurt	½ cup
Pink salt	¼ tsp
Water	½ cup

For idli burger:

Lettuce	2-3 leaves
Tomato	1 no
Potato	2 medium size
Carrots	¼ cup
Spinach	3-4 leaves
Black pepper	¼ tsp
Pink salt	¼ tsp
Filtered oil	2 tsp

Method

- For the idli batter, soak the rice and urad dal overnight.
- Next day, strain water from the soaked rice and urad dal. Take a bowl, add the rice, urad dal, and yoghurt, followed by salt, and blend it in a food processor. Let it rest for 4-5 hours.
- Later, preheat the steamer on the stove for 10 minutes. Add water if required into the idli batter. Give it a good stir.
- Take a medium size bowl and brush it with oil. Add the idli batter into the bowl and let it steam for about 15 minutes.
- After 15 minutes, remove the idli and slit it from between to give it a bun shape.
- For the burger patty, place a dekchi on a stove, fill it with water and bring it to boil.
- Add spinach to the boiling water and boil for 2-3 minutes. Rinse the spinach under cool, running water.
- Make a smooth paste of the boiled spinach in a blender.
- In the same dekchi filled with boiled water, add the carrots and boil them till they get tender. Later, strain the vegetables.
- Place a pressure cooker on the stove and add the potatoes into it. Seal the pressure cooker and let them cook until 3 whistles.
- Let the pressure cooker cool down and remove the potatoes. Mash the potatoes, carrots and spinach into a paste. Shape into medium-size patties.
- Place a tawa on the stove, add some oil and place the patties. Let them cook until brown on both sides.
- For serving, slice the tomatoes. Place one half of an idli as the base. Then add the lettuce leaves, followed by the tomatoes. Add the spinach patty and cover with the remaining idli layer.
- Fix the burger with a skewer to keep the layers in place (optional).
- The idli burger can be served with fresh mint chutney.

Healthy cooking tips

- Avoid using excessive oil while frying.

- A good alternative to white rice is brown rice.
- Wash vegetables before cooking.
- Soak the dal for at least 6-8 hrs.
- Consume urad dal only in the afternoon. Soak it overnight and discard the water because it causes flatulence.

೪

INSTANT WRAP

Tempting, easy-to-eat wrap bursting with exciting colourful vegetables.

Skill level	Easy
Serving size	2
Place of origin	California
Season most suited for consumption	All seasons
Rich in nutrients	Carbohydrates, Vitamin A

Know your nutrition

Yoghurt: Curd is rich in lactococcus lactis, which encourages the growth of healthy gut flora and promotes digestion. It improves skeletal muscle since it is rich in calcium content and it is a good probiotic food the and prevents harmful microorganisms. The bioactive protein in curd reduces blood pressure and cholesterol levels.

Cabbage (Patta Gobhi): Cabbage is a rich source of antioxidant as it contains polyphenols and vitamin C, which lowers the risk of cancer and protects the body from free radicals. It has a high content of water and is also rich in potassium and manganese. It is a good source of high fiber that provides fullness to the stomach and lowers the blood cholesterol level.

Pepper (Miri): It is an important antioxidant in cognitive brain functioning as an antidepressant, boosting nutrient absorption and improving GI functionality. Its free radical-scavenging activity might help control the progression of tumor growth. Charak Samhita states its use in curing abdominal disorders.

Favourable for conditions

Athletes, Children, Adolescents, Pregnancy, Bone, and Muscle health

Calorie count

Serving size	Energy (Kcal)	Carbohydrates (gm)	Protein (gm)	Fats (gm)	Calcium (gm)
1	123	15.4	4.1	3.8	121
2	247	308	8	7.6	242
Serving size	Phosphorus (gm)	Iron (gm)	Fiber (gm)	Omega-3 (mg)	Vitamin A (mcg)
1	87.3	0.4	3.4	16.9	345.9
2	174.6	0.9	6.9	33.9	691.9

Ingredients

Leftover roti	2 roti
Curd	¾ cup
Carrot, sliced	½ cup
Capsicum, sliced	½ cup
Cabbage, shredded	¼ cup
Pepper	¼ tsp
Salt	¼ tsp
Mustard powder	A pinch

Method

- Mix carrot, capsicum, cabbage, pepper, mustard, and salt in a bowl with curd.
- Heat the leftover roti on both sides.

- Put the mixture in the center of the roti and fold it from both ends.
- Serve immediately.

Healthy cooking tips

- Whilst steaming the cabbage, add a pinch of cinnamon. Do not cover the cabbage initially with the lid while steaming as it contains sulfur, which may cause flatus and bloating. Cut it and check for worms inside the leaves.
- Green pepper can be used as an alternative to red/yellow bell peppers.

꧁

OATS DUMPLINGS WITH CARROT CAPSICUM DIP

Oats dumplings are a fluffy, steamed dish that fulfils your cravings nutritiously.

Skill level	High
Serving size	8
Place of origin	China, South East Asia
Season most suited for consumption	All seasons
Rich in nutrients	Dietary Fiber, Vitamins A, Vitamin C, B-Complex Vitamins, Potassium, Iron, Beta Carotene, Antioxidants.

Know your nutrition

Oats: Whole oats are rich in antioxidants, and contain a powerful soluble fiber called Beta-Glucan. They can lower cholesterol levels and protect from LDL cholesterol damage. Oats can improve blood sugar control.

Bell peppers (Shimla Mirch): Bell peppers provide key antioxidants such as lycopene, beta carotene, lutein and zeaxanthin that protect the body from free radicals, and help reduce the risk of cancer, heart disease and neuro degenerative disease. They are also rich in vitamin C, vitamin A as well as a moderate source for vitamin E, vitamin K, manganese and potassium. They have high amounts of fiber that provides fullness to the stomach and decreases digestion-related problems. They also protect the eyesight and promote bone health.

Carrot (Gajar): They are a good source of vitamin A, biotin, vitamin K, potassium and vitamin B6. They improve the eyesight and immune function, provide satiety and prevent constipation. They also reduce the risk of cancer.

Favourable for conditions

Weight loss, Diabetes, children, Adolescents, Gluten free, Senior citizens, Eye disorders.

Calorie count

Serving Size	Energy (Kcal)	Carbohydrate (gm)	Protein (gm)	Fats (gm)	Calcium (mg)	Phosphorus (mg)
1	223	41.1	7.2	0.6	35	30.9
8	1790	329.1	57.8	5	280.4	247.5
Serving Size	Total Fiber (mg)	Omega-3 (mg)	Sodium (mg)	Potassium (mg)	Beta carotene (mcg)	Vitamin A (mcg)
1	4.7	8.2	215.7	86.2	308.2	80.6
8	37.6	65.7	1726.3	689.7	2466	645

Ingredients

Rice flour	2 cup
Oats	1 cup
Tomatoes	2 whole
Carrot	1 small sized

Red Bell Pepper	½ cup
Green Bell Pepper	¼ cup
Cabbage	¼ cup
Fresh beans	¼ cup
Spinach	¼ cup
Pink salt	½ tsp
Turmeric	¼ tsp
Garam masala	¼ tsp
Water	1 cup
Sesame seeds	½ tsp
Ginger	½ inches

Method

- For the filling, lightly roast the oats. Set aside.
- Finely chop all the vegetables and roughly chop the spinach.
- Put oil in the kadhai and place it on the stove. Add cumin and wait for them to crackle.
- Add all vegetables into the kadhai and sauté them. Add turmeric and salt accordingly to the taste. Simmer it till all the vegetables get tender.
- Add oats into the mixture and then minimum water into the kadhai. Let this simmer till ready. Add the chopped spinach to the mixture and give it a stir.
- Let the oats cool. Then squeeze out the excess water from the oats mixture with the help of a muslin cloth.
- For the dumplings, make a dough out of rice flour and add salt accordingly to taste.
- Preheat the steamer for about 15 mins.
- Roll out equal size balls. Lightly flour the dough pieces and roll out the dough into equal size circles. Repeat the same process with the remaining balls.
- To assemble the dumplings, add 1 tbsp of mixture at the center of the rice flour dumpling wrap.
- With your fingers, lightly coat the remaining edges of the dumpling with water.

- Pleat the edges to seal. Repeat with the remaining dumplings.
- Place the dumplings into the steamer and allow them to get cook over a medium flame for about 5-6 minutes.
- For the capsicum carrot dip, slightly roast the ½ red bell pepper and carrot on the stove on a low-to-medium flame.
- Grind the vegetables in a food processor and add the sesame seeds to the sauce to make a thick consistency.
- Serve the dipping sauce with the hot oats rice flour dumplings.

Healthy cooking tips

- Use cool water or oil while folding the dumplings.
- Use steel-cut rolled oats and not processed oats or instant oats.
- If used as a powder, the oats should be nicely dry roasted before powdering.
- Wash all the vegetables before using.
- Avoid over-roasting of carrot and capsicum.

❧

PUMPKIN-ZUCCHINI-GOURD SAVOURY CAKE

Appealing savoury cake of exciting vegetables such as pumpkin, yellow zucchini and bottle gourd, which are rich in nutrients.

Skill level	Moderate
Serving size	4
Place of origin	England
Season most suited for consumption	All seasons
Rich in nutrients	Protein, Fiber, Vitamin A, Iron, Calcium, Potassium, Folate, Antioxidants

Know your nutrition

Pumpkin (Kaddu): Pumpkin has a antioxidant content such as beta carotene that protects the body from free radicals. It is also rich in vitamin A that helps in improving the eyesight and is a good source of vitamin C and E, iron, potassium and folate. It has a high water content and also has high amounts of fiber that provides satiety and decreases digestion-related problems. It also augments immunity and promotes eye health.

Zucchini: Zucchinis are less in calories and contains small amounts of iron, calcium, zinc, and several other B vitamins. It is a rich source of vitamins A and C, which support your vision and immune system. They also have antioxidant compounds such as lutein, zeaxanthin and beta carotene, which protect the body from free radicals, cancer and heart problems. They also promote skin health.

Bottle gourd (Lauki): Bottle gourd is a modest source of vitamin C, which is one of the most powerful antioxidants. It helps the body to fight against the free radicals, cancer and inflammation. It is even a good source of calcium and has a high water content. It is rich in dietary fiber that helps in curing indigestion and constipation.

Favourable for conditions

Weight loss, Diabetes, Children, Adolescents, Gluten free, Senior Citizens, Eye and Skin Disease

Calorie count

Serving Size	Energy (Kcal)	Carbohydrate (gm)	Protein (gm)	Fats (gm)	Calcium (mg)	Phosphorus (mg)
1	171	22.2	5.8	2.9	57.6	55.2
4	686	88.8	23.5	11.6	230.7	221.1

Serving Size	Total Fiber (mg)	Omega-3 (mg)	Sodium (mg)	Potassium (mg)	Beta carotene (mcg)	Vitamin A (mcg)
1	3.2	23.6	440	169.1	17.5	5
4	13	94.7	1760.1	676.7	70.2	20.2

Ingredients

Handwo flour	1 cup
Yoghurt	½ cup
Grated pumpkin	¼ cup
Grated bottle gourd	¼ cup
Grated zucchini	¼ cup
Turmeric	½ tsp
Asafoetida	¼ tsp
Pink salt	

Method

- Soak the handwo flour with yoghurt overnight.
- Add turmeric powder, asafoetida and salt into the handwo mixture.
- Add ½ tbsp oil and all the grated veggies into the handwo mixture.
- In a tawa, add ½ tbsp oil and heat it. Then add mustard seeds and let them pop. Once they pop, add the sesame seeds and curry leaves into the kadhai.
- Later, add handwo mixture into the kadhai with the thickness of ½ inch. Cover the kadhai and cook the handwo mixture for 15 minutes or until crisp, on a slow flame.
- As one side gets crisp, flip the handwo and cook for another 10 minutes.
- Cut the handwo into squares and garnish it with fresh coriander. Serve hot.

Healthy cooking tips

- Method is similar to that of a Gujarati handwo.
- Alternatively, carrot can be used as a substitute for pumpkin and other gourds for bottle gourd.
- Bottle gourd is used in making salads and juices. It is a healthy vegetable widely used for weight loss. It is low in calories and can be cooked in minimal oil. The peels can be used to make chutney, causing zero waste.
- Pumpkin is used as a thickening agent. It can be used as an alternative for potato. Also, it is a good substitute for carrot as it contains carotene and lycopene.
- Avoid over-tempering of sesame seeds.

SPROUTED VEGGIE ROLLS

A tempting stuffed wrap recipe bursting with organic flavours and highly beneficial sprouts.

Skill level	Easy
Serving size	3
Place of origin	California
Season most suited for consumption	All seasons
Rich in nutrients	Protein, Folate, Magnesium, Phosphorous, Manganese, Vitamin C and K

Know your nutrition

Sprouts: Sprouts are alkaline, and hence can be consumed to balance the pH. They are good for diabetic patients. They are also high in protein.

Coriander (Dhania): It reduces cholesterol deposition by lowering cholesterol levels and blood sugar. It is good for digestion as it contains high insoluble fiber and reduces Urinary Tract Infection. It is rich in vitamin C and hence possesses antioxidants and vitamin K. It eases muscle spasms and flatulence.

Carom seeds (Ajwain): A spice for stomach issues such as indigestion, flatulence, diarrhea and colic. It aids in relieving respiratory ailments. It is used as a cleanser, detox, diuretic and antacid.

Favourable for conditions

Weight Loss, Children, Adolescents, Pregnancy, Bone, and Muscle health

Calorie count

Serving Size	Energy (Kcal)	Carbohydrate (gm)	Protein (gm)	Fats (gm)	Calcium (mg)	Total Fiber (mg)
1	210	31.3	7.8	1.5	62.6	7.7
3	630	93.9	23.6	4.5	187.9	23.2
Serving Size	Phosphorus (mg)	Magnesium (mg)	Omega-3 (mg)	Sodium (mg)	Beta Carotene (mcg)	
1	104.6	43.3	54.5	588.3	657.1	
3	313.8	130	163.5	1765	1971.4	

Ingredients

Mung, sprouted and mashed	½ cup
Matki, sprouted and mashed	¼ cup
Carrot	¼ cup
Ajwain	1 tbsp
Lettuce leaves	2
Rice bran oil	2 tsp
Salt	¼ tsp

Turmeric	¼ tsp
Amchur	1 tsp
Wheat flour	60 gm
Lime	1 tsp
Coriander	1 tsp

Method

- Make a dough out of wheat flour and water and keep it aside for half an hour. Roll into rotis and heat on a tawa.
- In a pressure cooker, add all sprouts, salt and turmeric, and cook them for 5 mins. Once cooked, keep aside.
- In a pan, heat oil, jeera and carrot. Once the carrot is cooked properly, add the sprouts mixture to it. Squeeze lime and add coriander. Add chopped lettuce leaves.
- Take the roasted roti and apply some green coriander mint chutney. Add 1 tablespoon of the above mixture and wrap it into a roll.

Healthy cooking tips

- Soak well for 4 to 5 hours.
- Wash well and then boil.
- Sprouting is preferable.

❧

SWEET POTATO COTTAGE CHEESE WRAPS

Enticing burrito offers the goodness of sweet potato and aromatic spices.

Skill level	Easy
Serving size	6
Place of origin	California
Season most suited for consumption	All seasons

Rich in nutrients   Beta Carotene, Vitamin C and
                             Potassium, Protein, and Calcium

Know your nutrition

Sweet potato (Shakarkand): It's rich in fiber, a good source of vitamins A, C and B6, potassium, copper, and manganese. It also promotes gut health. It is speculated to have cancer-fighting properties and enhances brain function. It also supports the immune system.

Cow milk paneer: Ideal source of protein for vegetarians that is easily absorbed in the body. It is rich in calcium and vitamin D. It improves digestion and helps in weight loss. It helps in preventing pernicious anemia.

Favourable for conditions

Athletes, Children, Adolescents, Pregnancy, Bone and Muscle health

Calorie count

Serving Size	Energy (Kcal)	Carbohydrate (gm)	Protein (gm)	Fats (gm)	Calcium (mg)	Folic acid (mcg)
1	213	39.4	4.2	2.2	20.8	5.8
6	1282	236.9	25.2	13.5	125.2	34.8

Serving Size	Phosphorus (mg)	Total Fiber (mg)	Omega-3 (mg)	Sodium (mg)	Magnesium (mg)	
1	89.6	4.7	15.8	311.2	27.9	
6	538.1	28.3	94.9	1867.3	167.6	

Ingredients

Sweet potato   200 gm
Wheat flour   2 cups

Salt	½ tsp
Filtered rice bran oil	2 tsp
Lemon juice	4-5 drops
Grated ginger	1 tsp
Black pepper powder	¼ tsp
Sunflower seeds	1 tsp
Lettuce leaves, chopped	1 tbsp
Cottage cheese (paneer)	25 gm

Method

- Boil sweet potato with the skin for 10-15 minutes.
- Once it has cooled down, cut in small pieces.
- Add grated paneer, ginger, black pepper powder, lemon juice, sunflower seeds, chopped lettuce leaves, and salt and mix it.
- In a separate bowl, take wheat flour, slowly add water and mix well to form a dough.
- Take wheat flour dough and make large balls of it.
- Take one ball and roll in a circular shape.
- Roast well on both sides.
- Now take the roti/wrap, add the sweet potato mix and roll it into a tight wrap. Try and seal the ends while folding so that the stuffing does not come out.
- Serve hot.

Healthy cooking tips

- It is very high in fiber and a replacement for potato.
- Do not roast sweet potato as it increases the dietary AGE; instead, steam it.
- When making paneer at home, try to use cow milk because paneer made from cow milk is lower in fat compared to that made from buffalo milk.

VEGGIE BUDDHA BOWL

A yogi's vivacious recipe with an abundance of all essential nutrients, vitamin, minerals and fiber.

Skill level	Easy
Serving size	2
Place of origin	China
Season most suited for consumption	All seasons
Rich in nutrients	Protein, Gluten free, Vitamin A, Vitamin C, B-complex vitamins, Vitamin E, Iron, Calcium, Manganese, Antioxidants

Know your nutrition

Tofu: Tofu is high in plant protein and contains all the essential amino acids your body needs. It also has a wide variety of vitamins and minerals. It is naturally gluten-free and low in calories. The calcium and magnesium in tofu helps to strengthen bones, lessen symptoms of premenstrual syndrome, regulate blood sugar, and prevent migraine headaches.

Cauliflower: Cauliflower is a rich source of flavonoids, which is an antioxidant that helps in reducing free radicals, cancer, heart disease and neuro degenerative disease. It also has high amounts of fiber, which provides satiety and decreases digestion-related problems.

Holy basil leaves: Lowers blood sugar, reduces stress and anxiety, improves your immune function by fighting allergies, beats inflammation as it contains volatile oil called eugenol, protects your blood vessels, rich in antioxidants that fights against bacteria and infections and lowers cholesterol.

Favourable for conditions

Weight loss, Diabetes, Children, Adolescents, Gluten-free

Calorie count

Serving Size	Energy (Kcal)	Carbohydrate (gm)	Total Fiber (mg)	Protein (gm)	Fats (gm)	Omega-3 (mg)
1	237	37.9	4.1	7.2	3.6	44.4
2	474	75.8	8.2	14.4	7.2	88.9

Serving Size	Calcium (mg)	Phosphorus (mg)	Sodium (mg)	Potassium (mg)	Beta-carotene (mcg)	Vitamin C (mg)
1	48.8	81.3	877.1	430.3	1048.1	7.4
2	97.7	162.	1754.3	860.7	2096.2	14.9

Ingredients

Brown rice	1 small cup
Tofu/paneer	75 gms
Sprouts	1 tbsp
Sesame seeds	½ tsp
Spinach	3-4 leaves
Carrots	¼ cup
Purple/white cabbage	¼ cup
Tomato	¼ cup
Olive oil	1 tsp
Pink salt	¼ tsp
Fresh coriander (cilantro)	to garnish
Lemon juice	1 tsp

For sauce:

Cauliflower	½ cup
Basil	¼ cup
Salt	¼ tsp

Method

- Soak the brown rice overnight.
- Rinse the rice well under running water.
- Julienne the carrot and cabbage and the spinach, tomato and cauliflower.
- Place the dekchi filled with water on the stove. Transfer the rice into the dekchi and cook it for about 30 minutes. Later, turn off the flame and cover the dekchi with a lid for 10 minutes. Then remove the lid and season the brown rice well.
- Place another dekchi and add all the vegetables and bring them to a boil. Later, rinse them under running water and strain them.
- Then, add the rice, tofu, and all the vegetables except cauliflower into a bowl. Season it well, add olive oil and give the mixture a good toss. Garnish it with fresh cilantro and squeeze lemon juice. Add sesame seeds as a topping to the mixture.
- For the sauce, add the chopped cauliflower and roughly chopped basil into the blender and blend it. Season it well if required.
- Serve it with the Budha bowl.

Healthy cooking tips

- Paneer can be used as a substitute to tofu.
- To prepare soft tofu, just steam the soya milk and it will get coagulated.
- Wash all the vegetables before using and avoid overcooking them.
- Good alternative to brown rice is black rice.
- Do not throw away the strained rice water. Use it in other preparations like soups.
- Avoid roasting of sesame seeds.
- Squeeze the lemon over the food once is completely prepared.
- Olive oil is ideal for minimum cooking time. Not recommended for traditional high-temperature Indian style of cooking vegetables.

VEGETABLE DUMPLINGS

An Oriental version of steamed and stuffed modak

Skill level	Moderate
Serving size	5
Place of origin	China, South East Asia
Season most suited for consumption	All seasons
Rich in nutrients	Magnesium, Protein, Iron, Vitamin C and A, Fiber, Potassium

Know your nutrition

Green peas are one of the best plant-based sources of protein, along with their high amount of fiber, which is a major reason why they are so filling. These contain a decent amount of heart-healthy minerals, such as magnesium, potassium, and calcium, and even regulate blood sugar levels.

Favourable for conditions

Weight loss, Children, Diabetes, Hypertension, Cardiac health, Senior citizens

Calorie count

Serving Size	Energy (Kcal)	Carbohydrate (gm)	Protein (gm)	Fats (gm)	Calcium (mg)	Phosphorus (mg)	Iron (mg)
1	183	27.6	4.9	1.4	29.6	8.1	0.8
5	916	138.2	24.4	7.2	147.8	40.5	4.1

Serving Size	Potassium (mg)	Magnesium (mg)	Total Fiber (mg)	Omega-3 (mg)	Vitamin A (mcg)	Vitamin C (mg)	
1	72.1	3.7	4	6.1	117.1	1.2	
2	360.4	18.4	19.8	30.7	585.7	6	

Ingredients

Rice flour	1 cup
Water	1 cup
Carrot	½ cup
Cabbage	½ cup
Green Peas	¼ cup
Cumin seeds	1 tsp
Pepper powder	¼ tsp
Oil	1½ tbsp

Method

- In a pan, add 1 tbsp oil, cumin seeds, cabbage, carrot and green peas. Cook until soft.
- In another pan, add water. Let it boil. Add rice flour and stir it continuously. Make the dough immediately.
- Make tiny balls and roll them in a circular shape. Add the stuffing and seal it.
- Grease a steamer bowl with oil and place the dumplings. Let it steam for 5-7 minutes and serve it with any dip of your choice.

Healthy cooking tips

- Cut the cabbage and check for worms.
- Sautéing and tempering of cumin seeds should be done for a short time and on medium flame.

2. FRITTERS

BROCCOLI FRITTERS

Vibrant broccoli fritters with the goodness of paneer.

Skill level	Easy
Serving size	4
Place of origin	Southern US

Season most suited	All seasons
for consumption	
Rich in nutrients	Beta Carotene, Vitamin B9, Vitamin C, Calcium, Potassium

Know your nutrition

Broccoli: Broccoli is a good source of several vitamins and minerals such as vitamins A, C and B9, and zinc. It also has a good percentage of beta-carotene and lutein that protect the skin and help in relieving inflammation. It also helps in reducing cholesterol, blood pressure, and risk of cancer.

Cow milk paneer: Cow milk paneer is an ideal source of protein for vegetarians, which is easily absorbed in the body. It is rich in calcium and vitamin D. It improves digestion and helps in weight loss. It also helps in preventing pernicious anemia.

Favourable for conditions

Gluten-free, Children, Senior citizens, Pregnancy, Lactation, Digestive issues, Skin disease

Calorie count

Serving Size	Energy (Kcal)	Carbohydrate (gm)	Protein (gm)	Fats (gm)	Calcium (mg)	Phosphorus (mg)
1	126	8.3	4.3	5.6	111.4	23.4
4	505	33.4	17.4	22.5	445.7	93.7
Serving Size	Total Fiber (mg)	Omega-3 (mg)	Potassium (mg)	Vitamin C (mg)	Folates (mcg)	Beta-Carotene (mcg)
1	1.7	8.1	166.6	10.2	34.1	137.7
4	7	32.4	666.5	40.8	136.5	551

Ingredients

| Broccoli (shredded) | 1 bowl |
| Paneer | 1 cup |

Chickpea flour	1 tbsp
Coriander	1 cup
Lemon juice	1 tsp
Ajwain	½ tsp
Amchur powder	1 tsp
Salt	½ tsp
Oil	For greasing

Method

- In a bowl add all the above ingredients and mix well
- Divide the mixture into equal portions and shape them into small round tikkis.
- Brush a non-stick tawa (griddle) with a little oil and cook the tikkis until both sides turn golden brown.
- Drain on absorbent paper and serve hot.

Healthy cooking tips

- Broccoli is a healthy and versatile vegetable. Wash the vegetable properly. If you want to steam it, do not overcook it as it becomes mushy, which also has an impact on the nutrients content.
- Add a pinch of salt while steaming; it brightens the colour.
- When making paneer at home, try to use cow milk because paneer made of cow milk is lower in fat compared to that made of buffalo milk.

❧

CARROT CHICKPEA FRITTERS

Mouth-watering fritters that are rich in fiber, vitamin A and essential nutrients—a perfect snack for winters.

| Skill level | Moderate |
| Serving size | 4 |

Place of origin	Southern US
Season most suited for consumption	Winter
Rich in nutrients	Potassium, Vitamin A, Iron, Magnesium, Fiber, Calcium

Know your nutrition

Chickpea (Chole): It is a plant-based source of protein, ideal for vegetarians and vegans. It is a source of zinc, folate and copper. It increases satiety and helps with weight loss. It also helps to control blood sugar levels and improves digestion.

Cinnamon: Cinnamon is packed with a variety of protective antioxidants that slow the aging process. The antioxidants in cinnamon help relieve inflammation, which can lower the risk of heart disease, cancer, cognitive decline, and more. Cinnamon also contains natural antimicrobial, antibiotic, antifungal, and antiviral properties. Its essential oils contain powerful immune-boosting compounds.

Cardamom (Elaichi): It can be used to treat respiratory and GI tract infections along with kidney and urinary disorders (increases the frequency of urination). It reduces all kinds of inflammations, even of eyelids, and antibacterial infections of teeth and gums. It is an antidote for both snake and scorpion venom and used to treat food poisoning. It is also used as a mouth freshener.

Favourable for conditions

Diabetes, Hypertension, Cardiac health, Tiffin snack

Calorie count

Serving Size	Energy (Kcal)	Carbohydrate (gm)	Protein (gm)	Fats (gm)	Calcium (mg)	Phosphorus (mg)
1	150	18.3	4.5	2.3	25	48.8
4	601	73.4	18.0	9.1	100.1	195.4

Serving Size	Iron (mg)	Total Fiber (mg)	Omega-3 (mg)	Potassium (mg)	Magnesium (mg)	Vitamin A (mcg)
1	0.6	4.0	330.7	103.2	12.4	145.2
4	2.3	15.9	1322.8	412.8	49.6	580.8

Ingredients

Carrots, chopped	½ cup
Ginger, chopped	¼ cup
Chickpea, cooked	½ cup
Cumin seeds	½ tsp
Coriander seeds	½ tsp
Black Pepper	½ tsp
Cinnamon, ground	¼ tsp
Cardamom, ground	¼ tsp
Salt	½ tsp
Flaxseed	1 tbsp
Oats flour	¼ cup
Oil	1 tbsp

Method

- Blend chickpeas into a smooth paste and add to the bowl.
- Grate carrots and ginger and crush the cumin, coriander and black pepper. In a pan, put oil add the crushed spices and shallow fry it.
- Add those spices to the bowl and add cinnamon, cardamom, salt, oat flour, and flaxseeds. Mix well and shape into a patty.
- Smear a pan with oil and cook the patties till they turn brown and serve with any chutney of your choice.

Healthy cooking tips

- Can use zucchini or bottle gourd instead of carrot.
- Eat chole only in the afternoon, because consumed at night may cause bloating and flatulence.
- Do not add soda to it whilst cooking to soften it.

- Flaxseeds should be eaten as it is or can be powdered.
- Ginger has lipid-lowering properties and should be added in day-to-day recipes.
- If oats are used as a powder in soups or curries, they should be nicely dry roasted before powdering.

3. HUMMUS

GREEN PEAS AND HUMMUS CHUTNEY

Delicious Middle Eastern hummus with the freshness of mint leaves and peas.

Skill level	Easy
Serving size	1
Place of origin	Middle Eastern regions
Season most suited for consumption	All seasons
Rich in nutrients	Vitamin K and C, Phosphorous, Folate, Vitamin B complex, and Zinc

Know your nutrition

Chickpea (Chole): It is a plant-based source of protein, ideal for vegetarians and vegans. It is a source of zinc, folate, and copper. It increases satiety and helps with weight loss. It helps to control blood sugar levels and also improves digestion.

Mint (Pudina): It gives a cooling effect, aids in digestion since it is rich in fiber, and relieves nausea as it contains rosmarinic acid. It is rich in vitamin C and iron; hence it has antibacterial, antifungal, and antiviral proteins that can prevent infections and fight harmful microorganisms as it boosts the immune system. It is widely used to treat headache, muscle pain (since it is rich in vitamin D and calcium) and respiratory issues.

Green peas: These are one of the best plant-based sources of protein, which is a major reason why they are so filling. Because of their high amount of fiber, they reduce appetite and promote feelings of fullness. These contain a decent amount of heart-healthy minerals, such as magnesium, potassium, and calcium, and even regulate blood sugar levels.

Favourable for conditions

Weight loss, Anemia, Diabetes, Children, Adolescents, Bone and Muscle health

Calorie count

Serving Size	Energy (Kcal)	Carbohydrate (gm)	Protein (gm)	Fats (gm)	Calcium (mg)	Phosphorus (mg)
1	270	28.3	9.6	9.7	222.1	126.6
Serving Size	Total Fiber (mg)	Omega-3 (mg)	Sodium (mg)	Potassium (mg)	Folate (mcg)	Vitamin A (mg)
1	10.5	83.6	1740.9	348.2	118.7	164.2

Ingredients

Mint leaves	20 gm
Green peas	50 gm
Chickpeas	30 gm
Sesame seeds	15 gm
Salt	¼ tsp
Lemon juice	1 tbsp
Olive oil	1 tsp
Cumin	1 tsp

Method

• Take chickpeas and water in a bowl and soak overnight.
• Next day, boil chickpeas in a pressure cooker for 15-20 minutes.
• After it has cooled down, mash them and make a purée in a blender.

- Take green peas in a bowl, and make a purée of the peas with mint in a separate blender.
- Add sesame seeds, lemon juice, cumin, olive oil and salt in a bowl add mix well.
- In a separate bowl, add chickpeas purée, peas purée and sesame mixture and mix them well. The hummus is ready to serve.

Healthy cooking tips

- Use raw green peas, especially for dips. Do not boil them.
- Use fresh mint leaves.

❧

SWEET POTATO HUMMUS

Enticing Middle Eastern sweet potato hummus that's rich in protein, fiber, vitamins and essential nutrients.

Skill level	Easy
Serving size	20
Place of origin	Middle East
Season most suited for consumption	All seasons
Rich in nutrients	Proteins, Iron, Folate, Phosphorus

Know your nutrition

Sweet potato (Shakarkand): It's rich in fiber, a good source of vitamin A, C and B6, potassium, copper, and manganese. It also promotes gut health. Speculated to have cancer-fighting properties and enhance brain function. It also supports the immune system.

Olive oil: It is rich in vitamin E and K that reduces the risk of heart diseases and controls weight. It also acts as an anti-inflammatory, reduces rheumatoid arthritis, releases joint pain and reduces the risk of cancer, prevents stroke, reduces the risk of Alzheimer's disease, maintains blood sugar, improves insulin sensitivity. It also has antibacterial properties.

Sesame seeds (Til): Sesame seed is a good source of calcium that promotes bone health. Magnesium content in seeds also helps to lower cholesterol and triglycerides levels. Vitamin E and other antioxidants in seeds help to maintain blood pressure. Sesame seeds are also a good source of vitamin B. Sesame seeds are low in carbohydrates and high in protein and fiber that helps to control blood sugar levels.

Favourable for conditions

Diabetes, Athletes, Children, Adolescents, Pregnancy, Bone and Muscle health

Calorie count

Serving size	Energy (Kcal)	Carbohydrates (gm)	Protein (gm)	Fats (gm)	Calcium (gm)
1	157	21.4	5.4	3.8	18.7
20	3158	429.4	108.9	77.7	374.7
Serving size	Phosphorus (gm)	Iron (gm)	Fiber (gm)	Omega-3 (mg)	Folate (mcg)
1	43.0	0.4	4.1	1.7	91.8
20	861.9	8.4	83	34.2	1837.7

Ingredients

Chickpeas	4 cups
Lemon juice	¼ cup
Olive oil	⅓ cup
Sweet potato	1 big
Black pepper	To taste
Salt	½ tsp
Sesame seeds	½ tbsp

Method

- Roast the sesame seeds until light brown.
- In the bowl of a food processor, combine the chickpeas, sesame seeds, lemon juice, olive oil, and sweet potato.
- Purée until smooth; season with salt and pepper.
- Serve with your choice of chips, crackers, and veggies.

Healthy Cooking Tip

- It is very high in fiber and a replacement for potato.
- It can also be used as a thickener.
- Do not roast sweet potato as it increases the dietary AGE instead steam.
- It can be eaten post-workout as it's high in carbohydrates and high fibers.
- It is commonly used for salad dressing.
- Ideal for minimum cooking time.
- Not recommended for traditional high-temperature Indian style of cooking of vegetables.

4. CRISPY SNACKS

AMARANTH LAVASH

Argentina style lavash with the goodness of amaranth leaves and sesame seeds.

Skill level	Moderate
Serving size	4
Place of origin	Armenia, Iran
Season most suited for consumption	Summer
Rich in nutrients	Fiber, Magnesium, Vitamin A, Calcium, Potassium

Know your nutrition

Amaranth (Cholai): Improves bone strength as it is a rich source of calcium that prevents demineralization of the bones and vitamin K that helps to produce osteocalcin. It also aids in weight loss and digestion as it is high in soluble and insoluble fiber. It is rich in iron which is a good source for anemic and is a storehouse of essential phytonutrients and antioxidants that helps to reduce inflammation in the body.

Sesame seeds (Til): Sesame seed is a good source of calcium that promotes bone health. Magnesium content in seeds also helps to lower cholesterol and triglycerides levels. Vitamin E and other antioxidants in seeds help to maintain blood pressure. Sesame seeds are also a good source of vitamin B. Sesame seeds are low in carbohydrates and high in protein and fiber that helps to control blood sugar level.

Favourable for conditions

Children, Bone health, Diabetes, Hypertension, Cardiac health, Immunity, Stress

Calorie count

Serving Size	Energy (Kcal)	Carbohydrate (gm)	Protein (gm)	Fats (gm)	Calcium (mg)	Phosphorus (mg)
1	53	8.6	1.1	1	30.5	27.3
4	214	34.3	4.6	4	122.1	109.3

Serving Size	Total Fiber (mg)	Omega-3 (mg)	Sodium (mg)	Potassium (mg)	Magnesium (mg)	Vitamin A (mcg)
1	1.5	19.1	110.2	9.4	9.1	178.5
4	6.1	76.5	440.9	37.8	69.3	714

Ingredients

Amaranth (rajgeera flour)	50 gm
Whole wheat flour	50 gm
Olive oil	1 tsp
White sesame seeds	½ tsp
Oregano	½ tsp
Salt	A pinch
Oil	1 tsp

Method

- Take amaranth flour and mix it with the wheat flour.
- Add salt and warm water little by little and start kneading the dough until crumbly.
- Add olive oil and knead further till it becomes soft. Cover it with a damp cloth and let it rest for 15 minutes.
- Preheat oven at 180° C and divide the dough into 7-8 equal size balls.
- Dust one ball with flour and roll it into circle as thin as possible.
- Cut the circle into 5-6 triangles and sprinkle the seeds and oregano on top.
- Arrange them on a greased baking tray and bake for 10-20 minutes or until light brown and crisp.
- Take it out and let them cool and serve it with tasty dips.

Healthy cooking tips

- Amaranth is a seasonal vegetable. Wash well and make sure that it does not have worms. It aids in weight loss and digestion. Steam the vegetable and do not drain off the water, instead use it for making dals or gravy as it contains many nutrients. Kale can be used as an alternative to Amaranth.
- Olive oil is commonly used for salad dressing and ideal for minimum cooking time.
- Sesame seeds can be used wide. You can just sprinkle it on food or salad and also make chikkis.

- Do not sieve the wheat atta, retain the bran.
- Use the Punjabi atta or Jadaatta.
- While sieving, remove stones and impurities but retain fiber.

❦

BEETROOT LAVASH

A succulent vibrant lavash with the blend of beetroot and garnishing it with exotic spices.

Skill level	Moderate
Serving size	4
Place of origin	Armenia, Iran
Season most suited for consumption	Monsoon
Rich in nutrients	Fiber, Magnesium, Vitamin A, Calcium, Potassium

Know your nutrition

Olive oil, (Jetun ka tel): It is rich in vitamin E and K that reduces the risk of heart diseases and controls weight. It also acts as anti-inflammatory, reduces rheumatoid arthritis, releases joint pain and reduces the risk of cancer, prevents stroke, reduces the risk of Alzheimer's disease, maintains blood sugar, improves insulin sensitivity. It also has antibacterial properties.

Pepper (Miri): It is an important antioxidant in cognitive brain functioning as an antidepressant, boosting nutrient absorption and improving GI functionality. It's free-radical scavenging activity might help control the progression of tumor growth. Charak Samhita states its uses in curing abdominal disorders.

Oregano: Oregano is rich in antioxidants, which are compounds that help fight damage from harmful free radicals in the body. It also reduces inflammation and risk of chronic diseases like heart disease, diabetes and autoimmune conditions.

Favourable for conditions

Children, Diabetes, Hypertension, Cardiac health, Athletes

Calorie count

Serving Size	Energy (Kcal)	Carbohydrate (gm)	Protein (gm)	Fats (gm)	Calcium (mg)	Total Fiber (mg)
1	54	9.0	1.1	1.0	7.9	1.5
4	217	36.1	4.5	4.0	31.8	5.9

Serving Size	Phosphorus (mg)	Magnesium (mg)	Omega-3 (mg)	Sodium (mg)	Potassium (mg)	
1	24.2	9.3	113.4	117.1	69.4	
4	96.7	37.4	453.8	468.3	277.5	

Ingredients

Beetroot puree	50 gm
Whole wheat flour	50 gm
Olive oil	1 tsp
Flaxseeds	½ tsp
Black pepper powder	½ tsp
Oregano	½ tsp
Salt	A pinch
Oil	1 tsp

Method

- Take beetroot puree and mix it with the wheat flour.
- Add salt and warm water little by little and start kneading the dough until crumbly.
- Add olive oil and knead further till it becomes soft and cover it with a damp cloth and let it rest for 15 minutes.

- Preheat oven at 1800 C and divide the dough into 7-8 equal size balls.
- Dust one ball with flour and roll it into circle as thin as possible.
- Cut the circle into 5-6 triangles and sprinkle the seeds and oregano on top.
- Arrange them on a greased baking tray and bake it for 10-20 minutes or until light brown and crisp.
- Take it out and let them cool and serve it with tasty dips.

Healthy cooking tips

- Raw beetroot has a lower Glycemic Index than cooked beetroot and is beneficial for diabetic patients.
- Beetroot juice helps to reduce blood pressure, improves metabolism, and exercise stamina.
- Olive oil is commonly used for salad dressing and ideal for minimum cooking time.
- Sesame seeds can be used widely. You can just sprinkle it on food or salad, also make chikkis.
- Do not sieve the wheat atta, retain the bran.
- Use the Punjabi atta or Jadaatta.
- While sieving, remove stones and impurities but retain fiber.

❧

FLAX SESAME CRACKERS

A healthy light wheat cracker with good quantity of sesame seeds and flax seeds.

Skill level	Easy
Serving size	6
Place of origin	Greece, Europe
Season most suited for consumption	All seasons
Rich in nutrients	Phosphorus, Calcium

Know your nutrition

Oats: Whole oats are rich in antioxidants, and contain a powerful soluble fiber called Beta-Glucan. They can lower cholesterol levels and protect LDL cholesterol from damage. Oats can improve blood sugar levels.

Flax seeds (Alashi): Flax seeds are a rich source of omega-3 fatty acids that reduces inflammation and risk of stroke. It also contains lignans, which reduces the risk of breast cancer. High dietary fiber content in seeds prevents constipation and reduces cholesterol level.

Rock salt (Sendha Namak): Rock salt contains various trace minerals such as manganese, iron, copper, zinc which is known to improve digestion and is a natural way to relieve stomach pain. Mineral baths are a great way to relieve sore or cramped muscles.

Favourable for conditions

Diabetes, Cardiac health, Athletes, Children, Adolescents, Pregnancy

Calorie count

Serving size	Energy (kcal)	Carbohydrates (gm)	Protein (gm)	Fats (gm)	Omega-3 (mg)
1	350	14.1	3.8	6	448
6	819	84.6	22.8	36.1	2688.1
Serving size	Calcium (gm)	Phosphorus (gm)	Iron (gm)	Fiber (gm)	
1	91.2	71	1.5	3.1	
6	547.5	426	9	18.8	

Ingredients

Whole wheat flour   ½ cup
Oats   ½ cup

Flax seeds	2 tbsp
Sesame seeds	4 tbsp
Rock Salt	½ tsp
Oil	1 tbsp

Method

- Grind the oats and flaxseeds. Mix whole wheat flour, sesame seeds, and salt.
- Add oil and knead into a ball and roll out. Make little rounds.
- Bake it in a pre-heat oven at 180° C for 20 minutes.
- Store in an air-tight container.

Healthy cooking tips

- It should be eaten as is or it can be powdered and added to dals and vegetables.
- It can be sprinkled over salad and can be added to smoothies, rotis, dals, mukhwas.
- If roasted in excess, its properties will change.

❧

OATS LAVASH

Light, fiber-rich easy-to-make oats snack that even fulfils the cravings.

Skill level	Moderate
Serving size	4
Place of origin	Iran
Season most suited for consumption	All seasons
Rich in nutrients	Fiber, Magnesium, Calcium, Potassium, Protein

Know your nutrition

Oats: Whole oats are rich in antioxidants, and contain a powerful soluble fiber called Beta-glucan. They can lower cholesterol levels and protect LDL cholesterol from damage. Oats can improve blood sugar control.

Black Sesame seeds (Kale til): Black Sesame seeds are a good source of calcium as they contain heavy amounts of protein, manganese, iron, copper and phosphorous. They are rich in calcium and zinc, which is also a good source of concentrated calories. Black sesame seeds can keep your bones strong and assist you keep off osteoporosis. The sesame seeds also provide the body with vitamin E, which is required for healthy skin. They are also taken as a preferable source of proteins. Black sesame seeds has strong aroma and really good flavour. At the same time, it's rich in fatty acids also. Black sesame seeds are rich in minerals and preferable dietary fiber item.

Favourable for conditions

Children, Diabetes, Weight loss, Skin disease, Bone disorders

Calorie count

Serving Size	Energy (Kcal)	Carbohydrate (gm)	Protein (gm)	Fats (gm)	Calcium (mg)	Magnesium (mg)
1	96	16.0	2.2	1.2	22.1	7.8
4	387	64.2	8.9	4.9	88.6	31.1

Serving Size	Phosphorus (mg)	Total Fiber (mg)	Omega-3 (mg)	Sodium (mg)	Potassium (mg)	
1	46.0	1.2	3.9	216.1	36.9	
4	184.1	4.8	15.6	864.5	147.6	

Ingredients

Oats (roasted and powdered)   50 gms
Whole wheat flour   50 gms

Olive oil	1 tsp
Black sesame seeds	½ tsp
Oregano	½ tsp
Salt	A pinch
Oil	1 tsp

Method

- Take oats and mix it with the wheat flour.
- Add salt and warm water little by little and start kneading the dough until crumbly.
- Add olive oil and knead further till it becomes soft and cover it with a damp cloth and let it rest for 15 minutes.
- Preheat oven at 180° C and divide the dough into 7-8 equal size balls.
- Dust one ball with flour and roll it into circle as thin as possible.
- Cut the circle into 5-6 triangles and sprinkle the seeds and oregano on top.
- Arrange them on a greased baking tray and bake it for 10-20 minutes or until light brown and crisp
- Take it out and let them cool and serve it with tasty dips.

Healthy cooking tips

- Use steel-cut rolled oats and not processed oats or instant oats; if used as a powder in a soup or vegetable; the oats should be nicely dry roasted before powdering, which can then be added to the preparation as a thickening agent. E.g.: dals and soups.
- Olive oil is commonly used for salad dressing and ideal for minimum cooking time.
- Sesame seeds can be used widely. You can just sprinkle it on food or salad, also make chikkis.
- Do not sieve the wheat atta, retain the bran.
- Use the Punjabi atta or Jadaatta.
- While sieving, remove stones and impurities but retain fiber.

SORGHUM OATS CRACKERS

A light, wholesome fiber rich crackers that are gluten-free and perfect to start the day with.

Skill level	Moderate
Serving size	3
Place of origin	Asian countries
Season most suited for consumption	All seasons
Rich in nutrients	Fiber, Calcium, Iron, Vitamin A, C, Magnesium, Potassium, Phosphorus, Folate

Know your nutrition

Jowar: Jowar is rich source of fiber, which helps in facilitate your digestion, manages obesity and regulates blood sugar levels. Jowar is also rich source of protein that helps in muscle building, cell regeneration and gives you a feeling of satiety. Jowar is packed with various minerals and vitamins that help in keeping body healthy.

Rosemary: It is rich in iron, calcium, vitamin B6, A and C. It acts as an anti-inflammatory and anti-tumor agent and helps to boost the immune system. It is also used to solve digestion problems, including heartburn, intestinal gas, liver and gallbladder complaints, and loss of appetite. It also helps improve memory performance and quality. It is also known to boost alertness, intelligence, and focus. The aroma of rosemary has been linked to improving mood, clearing the mind, and relieving stress for those with chronic anxiety. It promotes hair growth, protect skin cells from damage and also fights against bacterial infections.

Parsley: It is naturally diuretic hence helps fight kidney stones and UTI. It is antibacterial and antifungal, which prevents infection and plays an important role in defense mechanisms as it contains good amounts of vitamin A and C hence has good antioxidant properties and protects cells by reducing the ageing process. It can reduce the risk of cancer as it contains high levels of a flavonoid called apigenin.

Favourable for conditions

Digestion, Diabetes, Hypertension, Cardiac health, Immunity, Stress

Calorie count

Serving Size	Energy (Kcal)	Fats (gm)	Protein (gm)	Carbohydrate (gm)	Calcium (mg)	Phosphorus (mg)	Iron (mg)
1	180	5.3	15.2	23.3	134.2	98.6	2.2
3	540	16	15.2	70	402.7	295.7	6.6

Serving Size	Total Fiber (mg)	Omega-3 (mg)	Potassium (mg)	Magnesium (mg)	Vitamin A (mcg)	Vitamin C (mg)	Folate (mcg)
1	3.4	17.2	96.3	26.7	8.2	1	15.9
3	10.1	51.5	288.8	80	24.6	2.9	47.7

Ingredients

Sorghum (Jowar) flour	50 gm
Oats flour	50 gm
Thyme	1 tsp
Rosemary	1 tsp
Parsley	1 tsp
Sesame seeds	3 tbsp
Salt	¼ tsp

Method

- Knead the jowar flour separately with water and add dry herbs and salt.
- Knead the oats flour separately with water and add dry herbs, sesame seeds and salt.

- Roll out into rotis and cut lengthwise into a cracker shape. Then put them on pan and cook them till crispy and brown from both sides.
- Serve with dips, chutneys of your choice.

Healthy cooking tips

- Jowar is a good gluten-free replacement to the calorie-dense refined flour and it is very versatile and can be used in roti, bhakri, muthiya, etc.; ideal for IBS.
- Oats used as a powder in a soup or vegetable; the oats should be nicely dry roasted before powdering, which can then be added to the preparation as a thickening agent. E.g.: dals and soups.
- Thyme, rosemary and parsley should be added at the end of the cooking since heat can easily cause a loss of their delicious flavour.

✿

SPINACH LAVASH WITH BABA GHANOUSH

Spinach Lavash paired with healthy baba ghanoush dip from the middle eastern region.

Skill level	Easy
Serving size	4
Place of origin	Middle eastern region
Season most suited for consumption	All seasons
Rich in nutrients	Dietary Fiber, B-Complex Vitamins, Vitamin C Sodium, Calcium, Manganese, Potassium, Beta Carotene, Antioxidants.

Know your nutrition

Spinach (palak): It is rich in fiber, which induces satiety and also aids in weight loss. It helps to reduce the risk of cancer as it contains anticancer agents and antioxidants such as flavonoids, vitamin C, E and carotenoids. It is rich in lutein and zexanthin that improves eyesight and vision and can even reverse blindness. It is a good source of calcium, magnesium, potassium, iron and folate. It is also useful to reduce GI disorders as it is rich in fiber.

Brinjal/Aubergines (Baingan): Brinjal has high amounts of phytochemicals called anthocyanins and other B-complex vitamins such as vitamin B1, vitamin B5 and B6, which are rich sources of antioxidants. It also has a high amount of fiber. It also contains a good amount of minerals like manganese and potassium, which reduces risk of heart disease, cancer and regulates blood sugar level.

Yoghurt: Yoghurt is rich in Lactococcus lactis, which encourages the growth of healthy gut flora and promote digestion. It improves skeletal muscle since it is rich in calcium content and it is a good probiotic food that keeps ecosystem balance and prevents the activity of harmful micro-organisms. The bioactive protein in curd reduces blood pressure and cholesterol levels.

Favourable for conditions

Weight loss, Diabetes, Children, Adolescents, Gluten free, Pregnant and lactating women

Calorie count

Serving Size	Energy (Kcal)	Carbohydrate (gm)	Protein (gm)	Fats (gm)	Calcium (mg)	Phosphorus (mg)
1	212	29.3	3.4	6.2	28.3	86.6
4	848	117.2	13.7	24.8	113.3	346.4

Serving Size	Total Fiber (mg)	Omega-3 (mg)	Sodium (mg)	Potassium (mg)	Beta carotene (mcg)	Vitamin C (mg)
1	7.7	47.9	853.3	429.4	290.5	1.7
4	30.9	191.6	3413.3	1717.6	1162.2	7.1

Ingredients

For Lavash

Wheat flour	1 cup
Spinach	1 cup
Pine nuts	½ tbsp
Pink salt	¼ tsp
Filtered oil	1 tbsp

For baba ghanoush

Eggplant	500 gm
Sesame seeds	¼ tsp
Olive oil	1 tsp
Lemon	1 tsp
Yoghurt	1 tbsp
Pink salt	¼ tsp
Coriander	¼ cup
Black pepper	a pinch

Method

- For baba ghanoush, split the eggplant into half and roast it on the stove for about 20 mins. Then, peel off the skin and mash the eggplant.
- Add sesame seeds, olive oil, pink salt, black pepper, coriander leaves, water into a food processor and blend it. The mixture should be thick in consistency.
- Transfer the mashed eggplant to the food processor and blend it. Add water if required.
- Transfer it to the bowl, add lemon juice and season it if

required. Place it aside to let the flavours marinate.

- When serving, garnish the baba ghanoush with some coriander leaves.
- For Lavash, place a dekchi on a stove, fill it with water and bring it to boil.
- Add spinach to the boiling water and cook it for 2-3 minutes. Rinse the spinach under running cool water.
- Blend together the cooked spinach and pine nuts.
- For the dough, take a bowl add wheat flour, pink salt, spinach paste and unfiltered oil. Knead the ingredients and make a soft dough. Cover and place it aside.
- Divide the dough equally, and roll out circular Lavash of equal sizes.
- Take a tawa and place it on the stove. Once the tawa is hot, transfer the Lavash on the tawa and let it cook on one side until brown spots appear.
- Later, flip the tortilla on other side. Applying pressure on the Lavash with the help of handkerchief, cook the Lavash until it gets crisp.
- Serve hot with some sautéed vegetables and eggplant baba ghanoush.

Healthy cooking tips

- Wash well and make sure that it does not have worms. Do not sieve the wheat atta, retain the bran.
- Use the Punjabi atta or Jadaatta.
- While sieving, remove stones and impurities but retain fiber.
- Do not use refined flour.
- Add other grain flours to make it a multigrain aata which is far superior in nutrition.
- Brinjal is a seasonal vegetable. Wash it before cutting.
- Do not roast the brinjal it reduces the nutrient present in it, also it increases the dietary AGE.
- Use tawa roasting as a cooking method for lavash instead of

using oven baking.

- Avoid over roasting of lavash.
- Use broth to prepare a smooth paste for baba ghanoush.

E. HEALTHY FOOD ON THE MOVE

1. DRY SWEET SNACKS

DATE AND NUT COCONUT LADOO

Simple, tempting ladoo rolled with stimulating nuts and dry fruits.

Skill level	Easy
Serving size	8
Place of origin	India
Season most suited for consumption	All seasons
Rich in nutrients	Potassium, Calcium

Know your nutrition

Cashew nut (Kaju): It contains copper and iron that support healthy blood formation. It helps to reduce blood pressure and cholesterol levels as it contains potassium, vitamin E, B6. It contains lutein and zeaxanthin, which act as antioxidants and are good for the eyes. It also has a good amount of protein, which helps in the recovery of muscle and tissues.

Almonds (Badam): Almonds are rich in antioxidants and also have a high amount of vitamin E that protects against oxidative damage. Almonds also help to lower blood pressure and cholesterol level. It increases satiety as it contains a good amount of protein and fiber and is also good for heart health. It also contains magnesium which helps to prevent diabetes.

Dates (Khajur): Dates contains polyphenols that protect against Alzheimer's disease and colon cancer. The high content of iron in dates prevents anemia. Dates have a low glycemic index, which controls blood sugar level. High content of fiber in dates prevents constipation. Calcium and phosphorus in dates improves bone health. It may also improve brain health. The date contains potassium, which lowers bold pressure.

Favourable for conditions

Diabetes, Athletes, Children, Adolescents, Pregnancy, Lactation, Bone and Muscle health, Travel

Calorie count

Serving size	Energy (Kcal)	Carbohydrates (gm)	Protein (gm)	Fats (gm)	Calcium (gm)
1	129	16.3	2.1	6.3	18.9
8	1034	130.9	16.9	48.6	151.6
Serving size	Phosphorus (gm)	Iron (gm)	Fiber (gm)	Omega-3 (mg)	Potassium (mg)
1	28.4	0.5	2.5	8	178.5
8	227.2	4.3	20.5	64.2	1428.1

Ingredients

Dates, chopped	1 cup
Almonds, chopped	2 tbsp
Pistachios, chopped	2 tbsp
Cashew nuts, chopped	3 tbsp
Ghee	1 tbsp
Desiccated coconut	½ cup

Method

- Heat the ghee in a broad pan, add the deseeded dates and cook on a slow flame for 3-4 minutes while stirring it continuously.

- Switch off the flame, add the almonds, pistachios and cashew nuts and mix well. Allow the mixture to cool completely.
- Once cooled shape it into round balls.
- Take a ball and dip it into the desiccated coconut.
- Serve immediately or store at room temperature in an airtight container.

Healthy cooking tips

- Dates have a low glycemic index and are high in fiber. It is also a laxative agent.
- It can be added as a natural sweetener to many desserts.
- Avoid frying, roasting, or adding any salt to cashew nuts.
- Cashew nut powder can be added to the gravy for increasing thickness and creaminess.
- Cashew nut milk can also be extracted and used as a milk alternative.

❧

DATES AND CASHEW BALLS

Enticing ladoo prepared with dates and crunchy cashews

Skill level	Easy
Serving size	4
Place of origin	India
Season most suited for consumption	All seasons
Rich in nutrients	Natural Sugars, Fiber

Know your nutrition

Dates (Khajur): Dates contains polyphenols that protect against Alzheimer's disease and colon cancer. A high content of iron in dates prevents Anemia. Dates have a low glycemic index that controls blood sugar level. High content of fiber in dates prevents constipation. Calcium and phosphorus in dates promote bone health. It may also promote brain health. The date contains potassium that lowers bold pressure.

Favourable for conditions

Athletes, Children, Adolescents, Pregnancy, Bone, and Muscle health

Calorie count

Serving size	Energy (Kcal)	Carbohydrates (gm)	Protein (gm)	Fats (gm)	Omega-3 (mg)
1	294	23.6	7.7	19	23.4
4	1177	94.5	30.8	76.2	93.8
Serving size	Calcium (gm)	Phosphorus (gm)	Iron (gm)	Fiber (gm)	
1	18.2	103.1	2.5	2.9	
4	73.1	412.5	10	11.9	

Ingredients

Dates deseeded	1 cup
Cashew nuts	1 cup
Cardamom powder	1 tsp
Ghee for greasing	½ tsp

Method

- Take cashew in a mixer and grind coarsely.
- Take deseeded dates and grind them to a smooth paste.
- Take a small kadhai. Add ghee.
- Pour the date mix and cashew. Cook for 2 mins. Take off the flame.
- Bind it into balls.
- Add half piece of cashew for decoration.

Healthy cooking tips

- Dates have a low glycemic index and are high in fiber. It is also a laxative agent.
- It can be added as a natural sweetener to many desserts.
- Avoid frying, roasting, or adding any salt to cashew nuts.
- Cashew nut powder can be added to the gravy for increasing thickness and creaminess.
- Cashew nut milk can also be extracted and used as a milk alternative.

MURMURA LADOO

Tempting puffed rice ladoo that's rolled in jaggery and enhanced with flavours from nutmeg.

Skill level	Easy
Serving size	5
Place of origin	Gujarat, India
Season most suited for consumption	All seasons
Rich in nutrients	Potassium

Know your nutrition

White rice: White rice is a good source of magnesium, phosphorus, manganese, selenium, iron, folic acid, thiamine and niacin and additionally, its low fiber content may help with digestive issues.

Jaggery: Jaggery is loaded with antioxidants and minerals like Zinc and Selenium, which help prevent free-radicals (responsible for early ageing). Due to richness in essential nutrients, it can help cure menstrual problems. Jaggery is rich in iron and folate, which help in preventing anemia. It also Boost intestinal strength due to its high magnesium content.

Nutmeg (Jaifhal): It helps to stop diarrhea (in low dose), detoxify the body, and stimulate the brain. It has antioxidant, antimicrobial, and antifungal properties. Consuming too much of nutmeg results in sudden attack, irregular heart palpitations and vomiting.

Favourable for conditions

Athletes, Children, Adolescents, Pregnancy, lactation, Bone and Muscle health

Calorie count

Serving size	Energy (Kcal)	Carbohydrates (gm)	Protein (gm)	Fats (gm)	Calcium (gm)
1	101	21	0.7	1.2	18.3
5	504	105	3.5	6.1	91.8
Serving size	Phosphorus (gm)	Iron (gm)	Fiber (gm)	Omega-3 (mg)	Potassium (mg)
1	17.4	0.9	–	0.8	85.3
5	87.4	4.9	0.4	4.1	426.9

Ingredients

Puffed rice	1 cup
Nutmeg powder	1 tsp
Jaggery	½ cup
Ghee	1 tsp

Method

- Dry roast puffed rice on low flame till it turns crisp. Keep aside.
- In a large kadhai, add ghee and jaggery and stir continuously on low flame until the jaggery melts and till it turns frothy.
- Turn off the flame and add the roasted puffed rice and mix gently.
- Prepare small ladoo when the mixture is warm.
- Store it in an air-tight container.

Healthy cooking tips

- Sprinkling nutmeg is beneficial and helps soothe nerves and coughs. It can be used in various foods as garnishing or can be added in concoctions.
- Great food to be carried during travel

❀

PEANUT OAT ENERGY BALLS

Invigorating peanut oats energy balls that's simple easy-to-make and nutritiously satisfy the cravings.

Skill level	Easy
Serving size	20
Place of origin	India
Season most suited for consumption	All seasons
Rich in nutrients	Carbohydrates, Magnesium

Know your nutrition

Oats: Whole oats are rich in antioxidants, and contain a powerful soluble fiber called Beta-Glucan. They can lower cholesterol levels and protect LDL cholesterol from damage. Oats can improve blood sugar control.

Peanut/groundnut (Mungfali): Peanuts are high in energy. It improves heart health and prevents gallstones. It contains niacin, which protects against Alzheimer's disease and cognitive decline. It contains a good amount of folate, which is good for pregnant women. The magnesium content of peanuts helps to reduce the inflammation.

Favourable for conditions

Athletes, Children, Adolescents, Pregnancy, Lactation, Bone and Muscle health

Calorie count

Serving size	Energy (Kcal)	Carbohydrates (gm)	Protein (gm)	Fats (gm)	Calcium (gm)
1	102	9	3.3	5.9	15
20	2035	180.3	67	119.9	301.6
Serving size	Phosphorus (gm)	Iron (gm)	Fiber (gm)	Omega-3 (mg)	Magnesium (mg)
1	32.8	0.6	1.7	269.0	10.4
20	656.7	13	35.9	5380.4	209.3

Ingredients

Peanuts	200 gms
Seedless dates	10
Old Fashioned Rolled Oats	3/4 cup
Flaxseed powder	¼ cup
Sunflower seeds	1 tbsp
Ghee	1 tsp

Method

- Lightly roast oats, peanuts, sunflower seeds separately.
- Grind flaxseed, peanut and sunflower seed to a coarse powder.
- Grind dates to a smooth mix. Heat the ghee in a broad pan, add the dates and cook on a slow flame for 3-4 minutes while stirring it continuously.
- Then combine the dates mix to the oats, peanuts, and sunflower seed powder.
- Take a scoop of the mixture and roll between the palms to form a smooth ball.
- Store it in an air-tight container in the refrigerator.

Healthy cooking tips

- Peanut itself contains a good amount of fat so while using peanut use less oil /ghee in the recipes.
- No sugar is added. Enjoy natural sweet flavours of the dates

❀

SUTH-PEEPRIMUL LADOO

A traditional quick home-made remedy for cough, cold, stomach gas and gives the richness of flavour from ginger and peeprimul.

Skill level	Easy
Serving size	2
Place of origin	Gujarat, India
Season most suited for consumption	All seasons
Rich in nutrients	Gingerols, Shagols

Know your nutrition

Suth (Dry Ginger): It has strong antifungal characteristics, which fight against yeast infections. It helps in digestion; research shows that ginger is successful in emptying the stomach faster. It improves memory power and enhances cognitive functions. It also inhibits cancer growth, as Ginger possesses anti-cancer properties

Peeprimul and dry ginger together increases the mobility of the body, according to ayurvedic text. Peeprimul powder is a folk remedy for colds.

Favourable for conditions

Infection (Cold, cough), Cancer, Digestive issues

Calorie count

Serving Size	Energy (Kcal)	Carbohydrate (gm)	Protein (gm)	Fats (gm)	Calcium (mg)	Phosphorus (mg)
1	73	8.9	0.09	4	8.3	3
2	146	17.7	0.18	8.1	16.5	6

Ingredients

Suth (dry ginger)	10 gm
Peeprimul (Ganthoda)	10 gm
Jaggery	10 gm
Ghee	2 tsp

Method

- In a bowl add suth, peeprimul, jaggery and ghee and knead it into a soft dough.
- Divide the portion and make soft balls.
- Eat one per day and store in the refrigerator.

Healthy cooking tips

- The peeprimul powder should be free from dust, stones or ant debris.
- The powdered dry peeprimul roots should be without any lumpiness.
- Check the expiry date before buying the packaged peeprimul powder.
- Peeprimul powder can also be stewed in boiling water to make herbal tea, to which honey is often added as a sweetener; sliced orange or lemon fruit may also be added.
- Peeprimul powder is often used as a spice in Indian recipes to flavour dishes.

TIL LADOO

A festive treat recipe that is simple and appetizing with crunchiness from sesame seeds and gooeyness from organic jaggery.

Skill level	Easy
Serving size	10
Place of origin	India
Season most suited for consumption	All seasons
Rich in nutrients	Calcium

Know your nutrition

Sesame seeds (Til): Sesame seed is a good source of calcium that promotes bone health. The magnesium content in seeds also helps to lower cholesterol and triglycerides levels. Vitamin E and other antioxidants in seeds help to maintain blood pressure. Sesame seeds are also a good source of vitamin B. Sesame seeds are low in carbohydrates and high in protein and fiber, which helps to control blood sugar level.

Favourable for conditions

Athletes, Children, Adolescents, Pregnancy, Bone, and Muscle health

Calorie count

Serving size	Energy (kcal)	Carbohydrates (gm)	Protein (gm)	Fats (gm)	Omega-3 (mg)
1	230	23.7	6.2	12.2	24.9
10	920	94.9	24.9	48.8	99.8

Serving size	Calcium (gm)	Phosphorus (gm)	Iron (gm)	Fiber (gm)	
1	237.2	103.9	4.5	4	
10	949.1	415.9	18	16.1	

Ingredients

Sesame seeds (til)	⅓ cup
Peanuts	¼ cup
Desiccated coconut	¼ cup
Organic Jaggery	½ cup
Cardamom powder	¼ tsp
Oil	For greasing
Water	As required

Method

- Dry roast sesame seeds, peanuts, and desiccated coconut in a kadhai on a low flame. Keep aside.
- When the peanuts cool down, crush them coarsely.
- Mix the roasted ingredients well and add cardamom powder. Mix well and keep aside.
- In the same kadhai, take jaggery and 3 tbsp water, heat on a low flame. Stir occasionally.
- At this stage, switch off the flame and add the dry roasted mixture to it. Mix well.
- When the mixture is still hot, start making ladoos from it. Apply some oil in your palms to make the ladoos.
- Store in an airtight jar at room temperature.

Healthy cooking tips

- Sesame can be used widely. You can just sprinkle it on food or salad, also make chikkis.
- You can boil the sesame and then make a paste to make tahini sauce where sesame can be used as a thickening agent in gravies. It is also a Mediterranean dip.

2. SAVOURY SNACKS

BHEL

Mouthwatering puffed rice recipe that's simple easy-to-make with addition of colourful vegetables and crunchy peanuts.

Skill level	Easy
Serving size	2
Place of origin	India
Season most suited for consumption	All seasons
Rich in nutrients	Fiber, Protein, Complex carbohydrates

Know your nutrition

White rice: White rice is a good source of magnesium, phosphorus, manganese, selenium, iron, folic acid, thiamine, and niacin, and additionally, its low fiber content may help with digestive issues.

Tomato (Tamattar): Tomatoes are a good source of several vitamins and minerals such as vitamin C, vitamin K, vitamin B9, and potassium. It also has a high content of lycopene, beta-carotene that reduces the risk of cancer, heart diseases, and neurodegenerative diseases. Rich in dietary fiber that provides satiety. It protects skin and promotes eye health.

Favourable for conditions

Weight loss, Children, Adolescents, Pregnancy, Bone and Muscle health

Calorie count

Serving size	Energy (Kcal)	Carbohydrates (gm)	Protein (gm)	Fats (gm)	Omega-3 (mg)
1	253	25.5	6.4	13.3	11
2	505	51.1	12.9	26.6	22
Serving size	Calcium (gm)	Phosphorus (gm)	Iron (gm)	Fiber (gm)	
1	16.6	49.4	1.1	2.6	
2	33.3	98.9	2.3	5.3	

Ingredients

Puffed rice	1 ½ cup
Tomato	1 medium
Capsicum	1 small
Amchur powder	½ tsp
Rock Salt	¼ tsp
Lemon juice	1 tbsp
Roasted peanuts	2 tbsp
Sev	¼ cup

Method

- Mix tomato, capsicum, amchur powder, salt, peanuts, and lemon juice.
- Add puffed rice and sev and mix well.
- Serve immediately.

Healthy cooking tips

- Sprouted peanuts or boiled peanuts can be used.
- Sprouted mung can also increase protein content.

HEALTHY ROASTED MIXED SEEDS

Simple and healthful way to incorporate beneficial seeds in the routine.

Skill level	Easy
Serving size	20
Place of origin	India
Season most suited for consumption	All seasons
Rich in nutrients	Calcium, Phosphorus, Omega 3

Know your nutrition

Sesame seeds (Til): Sesame seed is a good source of calcium that promotes bone health. The magnesium content in seeds also helps to lower cholesterol and triglycerides levels. Vitamin E and other antioxidants in seeds help to maintain blood pressure. Sesame seeds are also a good source of vitamin B. Sesame seeds are low in carbohydrates and high in protein and fiber, which helps to control blood sugar level.

Sunflower seeds (Surajmukhi Ke Beej): Sunflower seeds are high in vitamin E and selenium, which helps to prevent cancer. And reduce inflammation. High amounts of vitamin E, magnesium, and omega fatty acid helps to reduce cholesterol and blood pressure. Chlorogenic acid in sunflower seeds may help to reduce blood sugar levels.

Pumpkin seeds (Kaddu Ke Beej): Antioxidants in pumpkin seeds reduce the risk of cancer, fight infection and reduce inflammation. Pumpkin seeds improve prostate and bladder health. The high content of magnesium helps to lower blood pressure and reduce the risk of heart disease. Magnesium also helps to control blood sugar levels. Pumpkin seed contains tryptophan which helps to improve sleep. The high fiber content in seeds helps to prevent constipation.

Favourable for conditions

Weight loss, PCOS, Cardiac health, Diabetes, Athletes, Children, Adolescents, Pregnancy, Bone and Muscle health.

Calorie count

Serving size	Energy (Kcal)	Carbohydrates (gm)	Protein (gm)	Fats (gm)	Omega-3 (mg)
1	27	0.4	1.1	2.2	136.6
20	544	9.1	22.6	45.2	2733.9
Serving size	Calcium (gm)	Phosphorus (gm)	Iron (gm)	Fiber (gm)	
1	20.9	11.1	0.4	0.6	
20	418.8	223.8	8.4	12.7	

Ingredients

Sunflower seeds	¼ cup
Pumpkin seeds	¼ cup
Flax seeds	¼ cup
White sesame seeds	1/8 cup
Black sesame seeds	1/8 cup

Method

- Take a heavy-bottomed pan. Add pumpkin seeds to it. Keep it on low flame and roast the seeds. Keep stirring occasionally. When the seeds start popping up and there is a roasted aroma, remove the seeds from the pan. Repeat the process with other seeds as well.
- When all the seeds are roasted, mix them all. Allow them to cool. Store them in an airtight container.

Healthy cooking tips

- Eat 1 tsp as a mukhwas or mix with other nuts and dry fruits to be consumed as a snack.

POWER-PACKED SEEDS

Revitalizing ladoo packed with natural sweetness from black dates and blend of beneficial seeds.

Skill level	Easy
Serving size	4
Place of origin	India
Season most suited for consumption	All seasons
Rich in nutrients	Calcium

Know your nutrition

Sunflower seeds (Surajmukhi Ke Beej): Sunflower seeds are high in Vitamin E and selenium, which helps to prevent cancer and also reduces inflammation. High amounts of Vitamin E, magnesium, and omega fatty acid helps to reduce cholesterol and blood pressure. Chlorogenic acid in sunflower seeds may help to reduce blood sugar levels.

Pumpkin seeds (Kaddu Ke Beej): Antioxidants in pumpkin seeds reduce the risk of cancer, fight infection and reduce inflammation. Pumpkin seeds improve prostate and bladder health. The high content of magnesium helps to lower blood pressure and reduce the risk of heart disease. Magnesium also helps to control blood sugar levels. Pumpkin seed contains tryptophan, which helps to improve sleep. The high fiber content in seeds helps to prevent constipation.

Favourable for conditions

Athletes, Children, Adolescents, Pregnancy, Lactation, Bone and Muscle health.

Calorie count

Serving size	Energy (Kcal)	Carbohydrates (gm)	Protein (gm)	Fats (gm)	Omega-3 (mg)
1	279	40.6	6	9.5	9.2
4	1116	162.7	24.2	38.2	36.9
Serving size	Calcium (gm)	Phosphorus (gm)	Iron (gm)	Fiber (gm)	
1	57.1	63.2	1.4	5.9	
4	228.5	252.9	5.6	23.7	

Ingredients

Black dates	2 cup, deseeded
Poppy seeds	2 tsp
Sunflower seeds	½ cup, chopped
Pumpkins seeds	½ cup, chopped

Method

- Grind dates. In a pan add ghee, grinded dates, sunflower seeds, and pumpkin seeds and lightly cook on a slow flame till 5 minutes.
- Once the mixture cools down, roll it and dust it with poppy seeds so that the seeds stick to the surface.
- Put it in the refrigerator for 2 hours and then cut into rolls in thin disks.

Healthy cooking tips

- Consumed in its natural form. Avoid adding additional sugar.

3. INTERNATIONAL TRAVEL SNACKS

NUTTY PRALINES

Satisfying crunchy nuts and seeds pralines with the native flavours.

Skill level	Easy
Serving size	4
Place of origin	South Asia
Season most suited for consumption	All seasons
Rich in nutrients	Copper, Magnesium, Protein

Know your nutrition

Sesame seeds (Til): Sesame seed is a good source of calcium that promotes bone health. The magnesium content in seeds also helps to lower cholesterol and triglycerides levels. Vitamin E and other antioxidants in seeds help to maintain blood pressure. Sesame seeds are also a good source of vitamin B. Sesame seeds are low in carbohydrates and high in protein and fiber, which helps to control blood sugar level.

Favourable for conditions

Athletes, Children, Adolescents, Pregnancy, Bone, and Muscle health

Calorie count

Serving size	Energy (Kcal)	Carbohydrates (gm)	Protein (gm)	Fats (gm)	Calcium (gm)	Phosphorus (gm)
1	297	24	6.9	16.1	249.2	119.8
4	1079	96.1	27.8	64.7	996.9	479.5

Serving size	Iron (gm)	Magnesium (mg)	Omega-3 (mg)	Fiber (gm)	Copper (mg)	
1	4.7	52.8	34.0	4.8	0.4	
4	19	211.3	136.2	19.3	1.7	

Ingredients

Sesame seeds	½ cup
Almonds	¼ cup chopped
Pistachios	¼ cup chopped
Ghee	1½ tsp
Jaggery	½ cup

Method

- Dry roast sesame seeds on a medium flame for 5-6 minutes. Remove and keep aside.
- Dry roast almonds and pistachios on a medium flame for 1 minute. Remove and keep aside.
- Heat the ghee in a non-stick pan, add jaggery, mix well and cook on a medium flame for 3 minutes, while stirring continuously.
- Add the sesame seeds almonds and pistachios and mix well.
- Immediately transfer the entire mixture on a greased tray in a thin layer.
- Cut into square pieces and allow it to cool.
- Serve or store in an air-tight container.

Healthy cooking tips

- Sesame seeds can be used widely. You can just sprinkle it on food or salad, also make chikkis.
- You can boil the sesame and then make a paste to make tahini sauce where sesame can be used as a thickening agent in gravies. It is also a Mediterranean dip.
- Have plain pistachio instead of salted pistachio.
- Pistachio can be used in kheer, halwa, or another dessert-like Baklava.

TRAIL MIX

A handful of nourishing mix of different textures of nuts and dry fruits.

Skill level	Easy
Serving size	4
Place of origin	Europe
Season most suited for consumption	All seasons
Rich in nutrients	Calcium, Phosphorus

Know your nutrition

Apricot (Khubani): Apricot contains a high number of antioxidants, Vitamin-C, A, E that fight infection and reduce inflammation. Vitamin A is also essential for eye health. The high content of fiber in apricot promotes gut health. Apricot also helps in lowering blood pressure due to high potassium content. Potassium also helps in maintain fluid balance and prevents bloating.

Favourable for conditions

Diabetes, Cardiac health, Athletes, Children, Adolescents, Pregnancy, Bone and muscle health

Calorie count

Serving size	Energy (Kcal)	Carbohydrates (gm)	Protein (gm)	Fats (gm)	Calcium (gm)
1	336	31.3	7.8	20.1	48.3
4	1342	125.4	31.2	80.7	193.3
Serving size	Phosphorus (gm)	Iron (gm)	Fiber (gm)	Omega-3 (mg)	
1	105.2	2.2	3.9	478.8	
4	420.8	8.8	15.8	1915.3	

Ingredients

Almonds	½ cup
Cashew	½ cup
Walnuts	½ cup
Black raisins	¼ cup
Dried apricot	¼ cup

Method

- Mix all the ingredients in a large bowl.
- Store in an air-tight container.

Healthy cooking tips

- Dried apricot can be used as a replacement of sugar in many desserts.
- Can be consumed as a snack with other nuts or tossed in a salad.
- Great travel food and munchy for office and school.

4

HEALTH BOOSTERS

Ayurveda promotes consumption of locally available food and ingredients. Seasonal, unadulterated, organic products, and green leafy vegetables are collectively known as shaka in Sanskrit, and they play an important part in the Sattvik diet.

1. **Amaranth:** It improves bone strength as it is a rich source of calcium that prevents demineralization of bones. Vitamin K helps to produce osteocalcin, aids in weight loss, and digestion as it is high in soluble and insoluble fiber. Amaranth has substantial iron reserves, a bonus for anemics, and is a storehouse of essential phytonutrients and antioxidants, which helps to reduce inflammation in the body.

2. **Bathua leaves:** These are anti-helminthic (kill parasites) as they contain fiber, heal wounds since they are rich in vitamin A, repair body tissues since they are rich in amino acids, contain a good amount of vitamin C, facilitating collagen production, and are known to be a 'heart tonic' since they are rich in magnesium and potassium. Bathua also helps in bone formation as it is a good source of calcium.

3. **Betel leaves:** They are used for the treatment of various disorders and are believed to have detoxification, anti-oxidation, and anti-mutation properties. Betel leaves' are

anti-diabetic, cardiovascular, anti-inflammatory, anti-ulcer, hepato (liver)-protective, and anti-infective. They are used as a stimulant, an antiseptic, and a breath freshener.

4. **Colocasia**: It helps reduce blood pressure, and maintains bone health as it is rich in minerals such as calcium. It has anticoagulation properties, is rich in fiber which aids in weight loss, and gives satiety. It is a rich source of beta-carotene, vitamins B and C, iron, potassium, phosphorus, and magnesium.

5. **Coriander**: It reduces cholesterol deposition by lowering cholesterol levels and blood sugar. It is good for digestion as it contains high insoluble fiber and reduces Urinary Tract Infection. It is rich in vitamin C, hence possesses antioxidants and vitamin K. It can ease muscle spasms and flatulence.

6. **Celery**: It improves heart health, lowers cholesterol levels, and reduces blood pressure since it is rich in magnesium, fiber amd potassium. It aids in weight loss, reduces bloating, and contains anti-microbial properties that fight infections. It has cleansing properties and has significant antibacterial abilities.

7. **Curry leaves:** They promote gastrointestinal health and help ease diarrhea, prevent diabetes, and reduce cholesterol since they contain a good amount of fiber and anti-diabetic properties. They prevent cancer owing to being rich in antioxidants such as vitamin C. They are rich in iron, and help in increasing hemoglobin. The leaves are beneficial for women who suffer from calcium deficiency, osteoporosis, etc.

8. **Drumstick leaves:** It reduces inflammation as it is rich in anti-inflammatory compounds, has antioxidant power since it is rich in vitamin C, quercetin and chlorogenic acid which fight infections, and helps in treating cancer as it is rich in niazimicin (an anti-cancer agent) that restrains the development of cancer cells. It also improves heart health by effectively reducing cholesterol levels, and improves bone health as it is rich in calcium and phosphorous which increases

bone mass and structural strength.

9. **Fenugreek leaves:** They lower blood glucose levels and blood lipids due to magnesium and antioxidants and are rich in fiber which gives satiety. They are the best source of iron, hence, recommended to anemics. They are also antibacterial and antifungal.

10. **Kale:** It reduces the risk of cancer, and improves immune function by helping fight allergies, autoimmune and inflammatory disorders. It improves eye health as it contains lutein and zeaxanthin that protect eyes and reverse blindness, and reduces blood pressure since it is rich in nitrates. It supports bone mineralization and prevents osteoporosis since it is rich in vitamin K, and aids in digestion and weight loss as it is rich in fiber and low in calories.

11. **Lettuce:** It acts as an anti-inflammatory agent that reduces inflammation, induces sleep as it contains lactucarium that acts on the central nervous system to produce pain-relieving and sedative effects, controls anxiety due to sedative and anxiolytic properties, and prevents cancer as it inhibits the growth of leukemia cells and breast cancer cells.

12. **Mint:** It gives a cooling effect, aids in digestion since it is rich in fiber, and relieves nausea as it contains rosmarinic acid. It is rich in vitamin C and iron. Hence, it has antibacterial, antifungal, and antivirus proteins that can prevent infections and fight harmful microorganisms as it boosts the immune system. It is widely used for headache and muscle pain since it is rich in vitamin D and calcium. It also helps relieve respiratory issues.

13. **Mustard leaves:** It prevents oxidation as it has antimicrobial, antifungal and anti-tumor activity. It boosts immunity as it has a good amount of vitamin C. It lowers cholesterol as it is rich in fiber, and maintains bone health. It prevents inflammatory diseases since it is rich in vitamin K. It helps in DNA duplication and repair due to the presence of good folate content.

14. **Parsley**: Its natural diuretic properties help fight kidney stones and UTI. It is antibacterial and antifungal, thus preventing infection and plays an important role in boosting bodily defense as it contains good amounts of vitamins A and C. It is a good antioxidant that protects cells by reducing the aging process. It can reduce the risk of cancer as it contains high levels of a flavonoid called apigenin.

15. **Radish leaves:** Protects the red blood cells (RBCs) since it is rich in iron. It is high on fiber, hence it improves digestion and regulates bile production. It protects the heart due to the presence of antioxidants such as anthocyanins, vitamin C, folic acid, and flavonoids. Potassium lowers your blood pressure and keeps blood flow in control. Vitamin C and zinc protect from common cold and cough. It also improves immunity. It keeps the body hydrated because of its high water content. It has skin special boosters to stay healthy, and that's mostly because of Vitamin C, zinc, and phosphorus.

16. **Spinach:** Its fiber-rich content induces satiety and aids in weight loss. It helps decrease cancer risk, its antioxidants such as flavonoids, vitamin C and E, carotenoids improve eyesight, and it is rich in lutein and zeaxanthin which protect the eyes, even reversing blindness. It is a good source of calcium, magnesium, potassium, iron, and folate. It also reduces GI disorders as it is rich in fiber.

Protip: In Ayurvedic texts, it is stated that chewing the twigs of certain medicinal plants such as neem makes the gums stronger, keeps your teeth clean and also exercises facial muscles.

Farming at home!

Microgreens, as we call them, are small, 2- to 3-inch leaves grown from seeds of vegetables and herbs. These can be grown in small areas in the house, in pots on grills. They are extremely nutritious and packed with phytonutrients. They grow fast, in approximately two weeks. The plants that can be grown are curry leaves, barley, wheatgrass, aloe vera, mint, jowar, ajwain, and basil, to name a few. These plants offer a nutritious addition to your daily meals.

SMALL WONDERS: SEEDS FOR A GOOD LIFE

These small wonders are known to be super-nutritious. Seeds are known to be a dynamo of nutrients and can be eaten regularly for a long list of health benefits. Rich in its nutrient profiling, plentiful fiber, fats, vitamins, minerals, and antioxidants, seeds are known to be extremely versatile and can be incorporated in many cuisines. With growing mindfulness, individuals are choosing to consume these seeds for enhanced health. They can help you lose weight while providing you with enough energy for the whole day. Oilseeds are important dietary constituents to combat chronic lifestyle diseases due to the presence of important dietary macro- and micronutrients.

1. **Sesame seeds:** Sesame seeds are a good source of calcium that promotes bone health. The magnesium content in seeds also helps to lower cholesterol and triglycerides levels. Vitamin E and other antioxidants in seeds help to maintain blood pressure. Sesame seeds are also a good source of vitamin B. They are low in carbohydrates and high in protein and fiber, which help to control blood sugar level.
   Uses: It is used to make sweets, chikkis, mouth fresheners, baked dishes and dressings, and sprinkled on Indian snacks like muthia, patra and dhokla.
2. **Flaxseeds:** Flaxseeds are a rich source of omega-3 fatty acids, which reduce inflammation and the risk of stroke. They also contain lignans, which reduce the risk of breast cancer. The high dietary fiber content in seeds prevent constipation and reduce the cholesterol level.

Uses: It is used in curd, as a mouth freshener, baked dishes, and dressings, sprinkled on salads, dals, and vegetables.

3. Watermelon seeds: Watermelon seeds are a good source of iron that helps to prevent anemia. The calcium content in seeds promotes bone health. Manganese, protein, and copper in these seeds are good for hair and skin health.
Uses: It is used in milkshakes, mouth fresheners, salads, energy bars, and as thickening agents.

4. Garden cress seeds: They have a high amount of Omega-3 that helps to reduce inflammation. A high content of iron prevents anemia and also promotes blood health. Garden cress seed is a galactagogue that helps in milk production in breastfeeding women. It also helps to treat nervous system problems as it has vitamin B2 and B6.
Uses: It is used in milkshakes, kheer, salads, parathas and as a mouth freshener. .

5. Fennel seeds: It is a good source of folate and iron, which are required during pregnancy. The fiber content helps to relieve constipation. Fennel seeds contain polyphenol antioxidants that reduce inflammation. Anethole in fennel seeds has an appetite-suppressing quality, which may help in managing weight. Anethole also has cancer-fighting properties.
Uses: It is used in detox water, mouth freshener, and in salads, parathas, dal, and vegetable preparations.

6. Chia seeds: Chia seeds have a high amount of antioxidants that have anti-aging properties. Chia seeds are also an excellent source of plant protein, which may help in muscle recovery. High fiber and protein content in chia seeds may help to lose weight. It has a high amount of omega-3 fatty acids, which reduce inflammation. Calcium, phosphorus, and magnesium in chia seeds promote bone health.
Uses: It is used in milkshakes, smoothies, sweets, detox water, salads, jams, and jellies.

7. Sunflower seeds: Sunflower seeds are high in vitamin E

and selenium, which help to prevent cancer and reduce inflammation. A high amount of vitamin E, magnesium, and omega-3 fatty acid helps to reduce cholesterol and blood pressure. Chlorogenic acid in sunflower seeds may help to reduce blood sugar levels.

Uses: It is used in milkshakes, mouth freshener, salads, energy bars, and baked dishes.

8. **Pumpkin seeds:** Antioxidants in pumpkin seeds reduce the risk of cancer, fight infection and reduce inflammation. Pumpkin seeds improve prostate and bladder health. A high content of magnesium helps to lower blood pressure and ' reduce the risk of heart disease. Magnesium also helps to control blood sugar levels. Pumpkin seed contains tryptophan, which helps to improve sleep. The high fiber content in seeds helps to prevent constipation.

   Uses: It is used in milkshakes, mouth freshener, salads, energy bars, and thickening agents.

9. **Fenugreek seeds:** Increase breast milk production and acts as a galactagogue, boosts testosterone in men, reduces fasting blood glucose and postprandial blood sugar, helps in controlling appetite, relieves heartburn and reduces triglycerides.

   Uses: It is used in curd, detox water, and spice blends. Soak overnight in water and consume early morning.

10. **Hemp seeds:** It improves cardiovascular disease by reducing inflammation and vasodilation. It also improves immunity, relieves dry skin and itchiness. It is a powerful source of antioxidants, reduces an inflammatory marker known as hs-CRP, is a great source of plant-based protein as it offers 25 per cent protein, and helps in weight loss as it contains fiber, which promotes satiety. It also aids in digestion as it is rich in soluble and insoluble fiber that delays hunger and GI transit time and reduce symptoms of PMS and menopause as it contains gamma linolenic acid and produces prostaglandin E1.

Uses: It is used in toppings, baked goods and protein shakes.

11. **Poppy seeds:** They improve the immune function as they are rich in zinc, and also rve function and bone health since they are rich in calcium. They reduce cancer cell growth and promote apoptosis, improve digestive health by preventing constipation and diarrhea owing to fiber richness, improve Type 2 diabetes and vision as they are rich in zinc, eliminate dandruff and facilitate the growth of shiny hair. They cure sleeplessness since they contain alkaloids that reduce cortisol levels and stress. They also improve female fertility by flushing the fallopian tubes.

    Uses: They are used in salad dressings, cakes/pastries, glaze, desserts, and porridge. Poppy seed paste is used in Bengali cuisines as well.

12. **Muskmelon seeds:** They contain antioxidants such as vitamins A and E, and help expel parasites from the intestine. They protect from cardiovascular diseases since they are rich in omega-3 fatty acids, and contain renal-protective properties since they are rich in phytonutrients. They also have analgesic properties and eliminate excessive phlegm from the body, offering rest from congestion.

    Uses: They are used in salads, smoothies, thickening agents and mouth fresheners.

ANTIDIABETIC	Sesame, sunflower, pumpkin, fenugreek and poppy seeds
ANTIOXIDANT	Sesame, fennel, chia, hemp poppy and muskmelon seeds
BONE and MUSCLE HEALTH	Sesame, watermelon, garden cress, chia and poppy seeds.
HEART HEALTH	Sesame, flaxseed, sunflower, pumpkin, fenugreek, hemp and muskmelon seeds
DIGESTIVE HEALTH	Flaxseed, fennel, pumpkin, hemp and poppy seeds

ANTI-INFLAMMATORY	Flaxseed, garden cress, fennel, chia, sunflower, pumpkin and hemp seeds
PREVENT ANEMIA	Watermelon and garden cress seeds
ANTI-CANCER	Flaxseed, fennel, sunflower, pumpkin and poppy seeds
GALACTOGOGUE	Garden cress, fenugreek seeds
SKIN and HAIR HEALTH	Flaxseeds, chia, poppy, watermelon and hemp seeds
ANTI-HELMINTIC and FIGHTS INFECTIONS	Pumpkin and muskmelon seeds
NERVOUS SYSTEM	Garden cress and poppy seeds

CHUTNEY: A DOLLOP OF GOODNESS

1. DAL-BASED CHUTNEY

AMBE DAL

A highly protein-rich Maharashtrian dal chutney with raw mango.

Skill level	Easy
Serving Size	2
Place of origin	Maharashtra, India
Season most suited for consumption	Summer
Rich in nutrients	Protein, Iron

Know your nutrition

Bengal gram: It is a plant-based source of protein, ideal for vegetarians and vegans. It is a source of iron, folate and copper and provides satiety and energy. It stabilizes the blood sugar, which prevents diabetes. It also contains phytochemicals called saponins that act as antioxidants.

Asafoetida: The Charak Samhita mentions it for treatment of respiratory, stomach and children's disorders, impotency, women's ailments, toothache and cholera. Its resinous gum is said to help patients of anemia, intestinal worms, aches and pains and fevers.

Carom seeds: A spice for stomach issues such as indigestion, flatulence, diarrhoea and colic. It aids in relieving respiratory ailments. It is used as a cleanser, detox, diuretic and antacid.

Favourable for conditions

Diabetes, Cardiac health, Bone health, PCOS, Pregnancy

Calorie count

Serving Size	Energy (Kcal)	Carbohydrate (gm)	Protein (gm)	Fats (gm)	Calcium (mg)
1	263	32.6	10.4	8	37.5
2	525	65.1	20.8	16	75.1

Serving Size	Phosphorus (mg)	Iron (mg)	Total Fiber (mg)	Omega-3 (mg)
1	91.9	1.6	7.2	90.2
2	183.8	3.2	14.3	180.5

Ingredients

Raw Mango, grated	1
Chana Dal	1 cup
Coriander	For garnish
Mustard Seeds	1 tsp
Hing	½ tsp
Salt	¼ tsp
Ajwain	½ tsp
Oil	1 tbsp

Method

- Soak the chana dal in water for 4-5 hours, drain the water and coarsely grind the chana dal in a mixer. Do not make a paste of the chana dal.
- Wash the raw mango, peel and grate it. Add the coarsely ground chana dal in grated raw mango.
- Heat the oil, add hing, mustard seeds and ajwain and pour it on the mixture of chana dal and grated mango. Mix the ingredients well, and add salt as per taste.
- Wash and chop the coriander and garnish the ambe dal.

Healthy cooking tips

- Raw mangoes are used to prepare chutneys and pickles or can be added to dals and pulavs.
- The water discarded post washing the dal can reduce bloating and as well as uric acid levels.
- Eat chana only in the afternoon, as if consumed at night, it may cause bloating and flatulence.
- Ajwain is great for digestion and can be used effectively as a post-meal mukhwas and to relieve bloating or flatulence.

2. FLOWER-BASED CHUTNEY

HIBISCUS CHUTNEY

An umami-flavour chutney that's enriched with vitamin C and calcium.

Skill level	Easy
Serving size	2
Place of origin	India
Season most suited for consumption	Monsoon
Rich in nutrients	Vitamin C, Calcium

Know your nutrition

Hibiscus flower: Hibiscus shows potential for cancer treatment and as a weight loss aid. Research suggests that the anthocyanins in hibiscus may hold the key to its anti-cancer properties. Hibiscus extract might have an effect on metabolism, preventing obesity and fat buildup in the liver. It is also useful in conditions like upset stomach and high blood pressure.

Coriander: It reduces cholesterol deposition by lowering cholesterol levels and 'blood sugar. It is good for digestion as it contains high insoluble fiber and reduces urinary tract infection. It is rich in vitamin C and K. It eases muscle spasms and flatulence.

Mint: It gives a cooling effect, aids in digestion since it is rich in fiber, and relieves nausea as it contains rosmarinic acid. It is rich in vitamin C and iron. It has antibacterial, antifungal and antiviral proteins, which can prevent infections and fight harmful microorganisms as it boosts the immune system. It is widely used for headaches and muscle pains since it is rich in vitamin D and calcium. It also relieves respiratory issues.

Favourable for conditions

Diabetes, Cardiac health, Bone Health, PCOS, Menopause, Digestion

Calorie count

Serving Size	Energy (Kcal)	Carbohydrate (gm)	Protein (gm)	Fats (gm)	Calcium (mg)
1	73	3.9	2.9	5	134.3
2	147	7.8	5.8	10	268.6
Serving Size	Phosphorus (mg)	Total Fiber (mg)	Omega-3 (mg)	Vitamin C (mg)	
1	50.3	2.6	41.7	3.1	
2	100.6	5.3	83.3	6.1	

Ingredients

Hbiscus flowers	5-6
Coriander leaves	1 cup
Mint leaves	½ cup
Sesame Seeds	2 tbsp
Chopped ginger	1 tsp
Lemon juice	½ tsp
Salt	¼ tsp
Honey	½ tsp

Method

- Wash the hibiscus flowers, coriander leaves and mint leaves thoroughly. Toss the sesame seeds on a hot pan and let them cool, then blend them with the hibiscus flowers, coriander leaves and mint leaves.
- Add chopped ginger, salt and a little amount of water. Again, blend them together to maintain consistency. Remove the chutney in a bowl, add lemon juice and honey. Mix well.

Healthy cooking tips

- To enhance the chutney's colour, blanch the flowers and then use them. Add the leftover water to the chutney.
- Mint leaves have a cooling effect, aid in digestion and relieve nausea. Also, they are used to make different detoxifying juices and salads. It can be used in the different recipes as it is a versatile vegetable.

3. FRUIT-BASED CHUTNEY

APPLE-GINGER-CINNAMON SAUCE

A classic combination of apple and cinnamon in a sauce with the infusion of health benefits from ginger.

Skill level	Easy
Serving size	2
Place of origin	India
Season most suited for consumption	Winter
Rich in nutrients	Fiber

Know your nutrition

Apple: Apples are rich in pectin and soluble as well as insoluble fibers, relieving digestive disorders. They improve heart health and cholesterol levels owing to the presence of quercetin and microminerals. They have a low glycemic index and hence provide satiety.

Cinnamon: Cinnamon is packed with a variety of protective antioxidants that slow the aging process. The antioxidants in cinnamon help relieve inflammation, which can lower the risk of heart disease, cancer, cognitive decline, and more. Cinnamon also contains natural antimicrobial, antibiotic, antifungal, and antiviral properties. Its essential oils contain powerful immune-boosting compounds.

Favourable for conditions

Constipation, Weight loss, Infection

Calorie count

Serving Size	Energy (Kcal)	Carbohydrate (gm)	Protein (gm)	Fats (gm)
1	106	18.8	0.5	2.9
2	212	37.6	0.9	5.9
Serving Size	Phosphorus (mg)	Total Fiber (mg)	Omega-3 (mg)	Calcium (mg)
1	5.9	2.8	20.9	9.3
2	11.9	5.6	41.7	18.7

Ingredients

Apples peeled and chopped, small	3 cups
Ginger finely grated	¼ tsp
Cinnamon	1/8 tsp

Method

- Peel the apple and cut it into small pieces.
- Cook the apple and grated ginger in a pan on medium flame for 2-3 minutes, and then add cinnamon.
- Now lower the flame, stir and cover for 10-15 minutes, till the apple softens and begins to crumble a little.
- If there is extra liquid, remove the cover and let the apple sauce cook for some more minutes.
- Remove from the flame and serve immediately, or put it in a container and store in a refrigerator.

Healthy cooking tips

- Cinnamon should be stored in a cool place and sautéed fresh. It should be ground in limited quantity.
- Freshly grated ginger increases the zest and prevents nausea.

❦

BANANA FLOWER CHUTNEY

Relishing Maharashtrian chutney recipe with the goodness of banana flower.

Skill level	Easy
Serving size	4
Place of origin	Maharashtra, South India
Season most suited for consumption	All season
Rich in nutrients	Vitamin A, Vitamin C, Omega 3, Folate

Know your nutrition

Banana flower: It is starchy and bitter in taste. It is rich in vitamins A and C, and can reduce the pain from burns. The extract of banana flower helps to prevent the growth of malaria parasites. It reduces the level of blood sugar and raises hemoglobin in the body as it is rich in fiber and iron, which assist in red blood cell production. It is given to lactating mothers to increase milk supply. It helps to cure excessive bleeding, maintains a healthy uterus, restricts constipation during pregnancy and promotes lactation.

Flaxseeds: Flaxseeds are a rich source of omega-3 fatty acids, which reduce inflammation and the risk of stroke. They also contain lignans, which reduce the risk of breast cancer. High dietary fiber content in seeds prevents constipation and reduces cholesterol level.

Favourable for conditions

Diabetes, Cardiac health, Bone health, PCOS, Pregnancy, lactation

Calorie count

Serving Size	Energy (Kcal)	Carbohydrate (gm)	Protein (gm)	Fats (gm)	Calcium (mg)	Folate (mcg)
1	84	1.4	0.5	8.2	5.9	7.6
4	335	5.5	2	32.7	23.5	30.5

Serving Size	Total Fiber (mg)	Omega-3 (mg)	Vitamin A (mcg)	Phosphorus (mg)	Vitamin C (mg)	
1	2.4	33.9	5.8	11.1	0.4	
4	9.7	135.6	23	44.4	1.5	

Ingredients

Banana flower	1
Grated coconut	½ cup
Peppercorns	½ tsp
Cumin seeds	½ tsp

Ghee	1 tbsp
Salt	½ tsp
Flax seeds	¼ seeds

Method

- Remove the outer peels of the banana flower one by one until the complete white center is visible.
- Chop the white portion of the banana flower finely. Add the pieces into a bowl with salt/turmeric to get rid of any bitterness. You can use all of the white peels also. Finely chop them and use them to make chutney. Allow them to stand in the water for 10 minutes. Decant all the water and keep the pieces aside.
- Heat a wok, add ghee, cumin seeds, peppercorns and flaxseeds and let them sizzle.
- Once the cumin seeds start to sputter, sauté them for a few minutes. Then add the chopped banana flower and sauté for a moment.
- Add salt, half a cup of water and cook it on a medium flame. Once the banana flowers are cooked through, remove from the flame. Let it cool completely.
- Once cooled, grind all the cooked ingredients with the grated coconut into a smooth paste, using only as much water as is required. We want the chutney to be thick. Transfer the ground chutney into a bowl.

Healthy cooking tips

- In case you don't want to steam the banana flower, chop it and soak in buttermilk until you want to use it. Buttermilk prevents the excess sap from sticking and avoids the flowers from turning black.
- Flaxseed should be eaten as is or powdered and added to dals and vegetables. Do not roast it too much, as excessive roasting changes its properties.
- Use salt towards the end of cooking so that it coats the surface

of the food, thereby requiring less quantities but enhancing the taste.

❀

GREEN MANGO CHUTNEY

A blend of raw mango, fresh coriander and grated coconut; a perfect blend most commonly prepared in summer.

Skill level   Easy
Serving size   2
Place of origin   Maharashtra, India
Season most suited for consumption   Summer
Rich in nutrients   Good Fats, Fiber, Iron

Know your nutrition

Raw mango boosts your metabolism, thus helping you burn more calories. It prevents dehydration. Raw mangoes are also high in niacin, which helps boost cardiovascular health. It is rich in antioxidants such as vitamins A, C and E, folate and fiber. So, it boosts immunity and improves digestive health. It also has a good amount of pectin so it can prevent cancer and cholesterol. It is a good source of energy.

Favourable for conditions

Weight loss, Diabetes, Cardiac health, PCOS, Pregnancy

Calorie count

Serving Size	Energy (Kcal)	Carbohydrate (gm)	Protein (gm)	Fats (gm)	Calcium (mg)
1	111	8	1.5	7.8	21.3
2	223	16	3	15.5	42.6

Serving Size	Phosphorus (mg)	Iron (mg)	Total Fiber (mg)	Omega-3 (mg)	
1	24.5	1.2	4.3	91.4	
2	49	2.4	8.7	182.8	

Ingredients

Coconut	25 g
Coriander	15 gm
Green Mango	1 small
Ginger	1 inch piece
Curry leaves	few
Mustard seeds	1 tsp
Oil	1 tsp
Salt	¼ tsp

Method

- Sauté mustard seeds, curry leaves and ginger in oil.
- Grind grated coconut, finely chopped raw mango and coriander and stir this mixture for a while.
- Lastly, add salt and grind it all to a fine paste.
- Add a tempering of mustard seeds and curry leaves.

Healthy cooking tips

- Coriander is a versatile herb used to make chutneys and garnish dishes. It is rich in antioxidants and can ease muscle spasms. It also reduces flatulence.
- Raw mangoes are used to prepare chutneys and pickles or added into dals or pulavs.
- Ginger has lipid-lowering properties and should be added in day-to-day recipes.

MANGO CHUTNEY

An appetizing recipe bursting with the tanginess of mangoes and blend of spices.

Skill level	Easy
Serving size	2
Place of origin	Maharashtra, Odisha, India
Season most suited for consumption	Summer
Rich in nutrients	Vitamin A, Vitamin, C, Folate, Iron, Fiber

Know your nutrition

Raw mango: Raw mango boosts your metabolism, thus helping you burn more calories. It prevents dehydration. Raw mangoes are also high in niacin, which helps boost cardiovascular health. It is rich in antioxidants such as vitamins A, C and E, folate and fiber. So, it boosts immunity and improves digestive health. It also has a good amount of pectin so it can prevent cancer and cholesterol. It is a good source of energy.

Jaggery: Jaggery is loaded with antioxidants and minerals like zinc and selenium, which help prevent free radical damage (responsible for early ageing). Due to its richness in essential nutrients, it relieves menstrual problems. Jaggery is rich in iron and folate, which help in preventing anemia. It boosts intestinal strength due to a high magnesium content.

Cloves: Its essential oils are traditionally used as a painkiller for dental emergencies. It has anaesthetic, antibacterial, antioxidant and antiseptic properties. It cures digestive disorders and has an appetite-stimulating action. Some Ayurvedic texts state that it can help subside cough, cholera, intestinal worms, arthritis, backache, blisters, boils, burns, sexual debility and morning sickness during pregnancy.

Favourable for conditions

Children, Adolescence, Weight loss, PCOS, Pregnancy

Calorie count

Serving Size	Energy (Kcal)	Carbohydrate (gm)	Protein (gm)	Phosphorus (mg)	Calcium (mg)	Fats (gm)
1	206	36.6	1.1	34.8	40.5	5.2
2	412	73.2	2.2	69.7	80.9	10.4

Serving Size	Iron (mg)	Total Fiber (mg)	Omega-3 (mg)	Vitamin A (mcg)	Vitamin C (mg)
1	1.8	3.4	94.9	12.3	18.2
2	3.7	6.8	189.8	24.6	36.3

Ingredients

Raw mangoes, peeled and sliced	2
Grated jaggery	3-4 tbsp
Salt	¼ tsp
Mustard seeds	½ tbsp
Kalonji	1 tbsp
Oil	1 tbsp
Cloves	3-4

Method

- Take raw mangoes and immerse them in enough water. Let them cook properly.
- Once they are cooked, add jaggery and stir properly.
- Add oil in a pan and add mustard seeds, kalonji and cloves. Pour this over the cooked mangoes.

Healthy cooking tips

- Raw mangoes are used to prepare chutneys and pickles or added into dals or pulavs.
- Sprinkle on salads, use as garnish, or add to rotis.

- Clove relieves kapha and are anti-microbial. It works best when tempered for a short period.

❧

SWEET AMLA CHUTNEY

A Maharashtrian chutney for winters with the goodness of vitamin C from Indian gooseberries.

Skill level	Easy
Serving size	2
Place of origin	Maharashtra, India
Season most suited for consumption	Winter
Rich in nutrients	Vitamin C, Fiber

Know your nutrition

Indian gooseberries: These are one of the most antioxidant-rich fruits. They have a high amount of vitamin C, which prevents the risk of cancers, diabetes, heart disease, and age-related illnesses of the brain. They have a high amount of dietary fiber and pectin. They are also rich in chromium, which helps lower blood sugar, cholesterol and blood pressure levels.

Sesame seeds: Sesame seeds are a good source of calcium that promotes bone health. Magnesium also helps to lower cholesterol and triglycerides levels. Vitamin E and other antioxidants in the seeds help to maintain blood pressure. Sesame seeds are also a good source of vitamin B. They are low in carbohydrates and high in protein and fiber which helps to control blood sugar level.

Favourable for conditions

Common cold, Cough

Calorie count

Serving Size	Energy (Kcal)	Carbohydrate (gm)	Protein (gm)	Fats (gm)	Calcium (mg)
1	172	23.47	1.44	7.9	59.5
2	345	46.9	2.9	15.7	119

Serving Size	Phosphorus (mg)	Total Fiber (mg)	Omega-3 (mg)	Vitamin C (mg)
1	35.7	4.4	71.6	113.4
	71.3	8.8	143.1	226.8

Ingredients

Amla	100 gm
Cumin seeds	1 tsp
Sesame seeds	1 tsp
Kalonji	1 tsp
Spring curry leaves	1 tsp
Jaggery	¼ cup
Salt	¼ tsp
Mustard oil	1 tbsp

Method

- Steam the amla. Once cool, deseed it.
- Grind the steamed amla in a mixer with a little water and make it into an even paste.
- Heat a kadai with oil, add the cumin seeds, mustard seeds and kalonji and let them crackle.
- Add ground amla paste and mix well.
- Add jaggery and salt, cook for a few minutes until the amla paste and other ingredients come together. Now, add spring curry leaves.

Healthy cooking tips

- Some amount of vitamin C present in the amla can be destroyed

while cooking or preserving but still, 1/4 the amount of vitamin C can still be retained so it can be used as a souring agent.
- Consuming amla in the winter season is important since the risk of getting infections is high in this season.
- Sprinkling of onion seeds adds extra nutrition.

4. NUT-BASED CHUTNEY

COCONUT-FLAXSEED CHUTNEY

Scrumptious coconut chutney recipe with the goodness of flaxseeds.

Skill level	Easy
Serving size	4
Place of origin	South America
Season most suited for consumption	All season
Rich in nutrients	Omega 3, Dietary fiber

Know your nutrition

Amchur powder contains many nutrients including vitamins A, E and C, and antioxidants. Amchur is also rich in iron and known to be quite beneficial for pregnant women. It improves the immunity system of the body and is also quite beneficial for your skin and hair. It is believed that amchur also helps in controlling your blood pressure as well as diabetes. Amchur powder improves your digestion and helps to fight acidity. Mangoes contain powerful antioxidants, which ensure good bowel movement and help combat constipation as well as flatulence.

Favourable for conditions

Diabetes, Cardiac health, Bone health, PCOS, Pregnancy, Lactation

Calorie count

Serving Size	Energy (Kcal)	Carbohydrate (gm)	Protein (gm)	Fats (gm)
1	107	2.3	2.7	9.7
4	430	9.3	10.7	38.6
Serving Size	Phosphorus (mg)	Total Fiber (mg)	Omega-3 (mg)	Calcium (mg)
1	32.1	4.6	1619.5	26.9
4	128.3	18.3	6478	107.5

Ingredients

Flaxseed	50 gm
Coconut	50 gm
Amchoor	½ tsp

Method

Using a mixer grinder:

- Grind all ingredients to a fine paste.
- Pour into a clean bowl.
- Add salt and mix well.

Best served with:
- As a part of a meal
- Rotis or theplas
- Wraps or burritos by adding cucumber
- Idlis, as a podi chutney. Can also be used to make idlis.

Healthy cooking tips

- Flaxseeds should be eaten as is or powdered and added to dals and curries.
- They can be sprinkled over the salad, and added to smoothies, rotis, dals, and mukhwas.

COCONUT-TAMARIND CHUTNEY

Succulent chutney recipe from South India that has a combination of flavours from coconut, tamarind, and native spices.

Skill level	Moderate
Serving size	3
Place of origin	South India
Season most suited for consumption	All seasons
Rich in nutrients	Good Fats, Fiber

Know your nutrition

Coconut: Coconut is low in carbohydrates and high in fiber, which helps stabilize blood sugar. It has an anti-diabetic effect due to its arginine content. It is high in antioxidants, which also prevents oxidative damage. It also has a beneficial effect on heart health and is good for skin and hair health.

Tamarind: It is helpful in diarrhea and has antibacterial properties due to the presence of lupeol, as well as anti-inflammatory and anti-nociceptive effects due to the presence of polyphenols and flavonoids. It protects the liver and cures fluoride toxicity due to the presence of antioxidants.

Cumin seeds: Ayurveda proves the benefits of cumin in the gastrointestinal, reproductive, nervous, and immune systems. It is antioxidant, antimicrobial, and chemoprotective to a certain degree. Cumin is also an anti-diabetic, antiseptic, a flatulence reliever, and a metabolic stimulator.

Favourable for conditions

Diabetes, Skin and hair disorders, Heart disease, Liver disease, Diarrhea

Calorie count

Serving Size	Energy (Kcal)	Carbohydrate (gm)	Protein (gm)	Fats (gm)
1	161	4.3	1.4	15.4
3	483	12.8	4.3	46.2
Serving Size	Phosphorus (mg)	Total Fiber (mg)	Omega-3 (mg)	Calcium (mg)
1	18.1	3.2	42.8	16
3	54.2	9.7	128.4	48.1

Ingredients

Fresh coconut	1 cup
Tamarind	2 tsp
Ginger	½ inch
Mustard seeds	1 tsp
Cumin seeds	1 tsp
Curry leaves	8-10
Salt	1 tsp
Water	½ cup
Coconut oil	1 tbsp

Method

- Put the coconut, seedless tamarind, ginger, and salt in a grinder. Add water and make a smooth paste.
- Prepare tempering with mustard seeds, cumin seeds and curry leaves.
- Pour the tempering on the chutney.
- Mix well and serve the chutney with idli, dosa or vada.

Healthy cooking tips

- Remove tamarind seeds before grinding.
- Coconut can be used in water, milk, or grated form in curries and gravies.

- Since coconut is rich in oil, minimum additional oil is required in recipes.
- Sautéing or tempering for long evaporates bioactive components in spices and reduces their efficacy.

❦

PEANUT CHUTNEY

Karnataka-style peanut chutney, which makes for a mouth-watering side dish.

Skill level	Easy
Serving size	1
Place of origin	Karnataka, Maharashtra – India
Season most suited for consumption	Rainy, Winter
Rich in nutrients	Folate, Niacin, Calcium

Know your nutrition

Peanut/groundnut: Peanuts are high in energy. They improve heart health and prevent gallstones. They contain niacin that protects against Alzheimer's disease and cognitive decline. It contains a folate in ample quantities, which is good for pregnant women. Their magnesium content helps to reduce inflammation.

Ginger: Charak Samhita mentions its uses in curing abdominal disorders, dyspepsia, nausea and vomiting associated with motion sickness and pregnancy, abdominal spasm, and respiratory, bone and joint-related disorders. It has an anti-inflammatory and antioxidant effect and, hence, boosts immunity.

Favourable for conditions

Diabetes, Cardiac health, Bone health, PCOS, Pregnancy, Lactation

Calorie count

Serving Size	Energy (Kcal)	Carbohydrate (gm)	Protein (gm)	Fats (gm)	Calcium (mg)
1	204	3.9	5.3	11.8	75.2
Serving Size	Total Fiber (mg)	Omega-3 (mg)	Niacin (mg)	Folate (mcg)	Phosphorus (mg)
1	3.2	15.4	2.3	3.2	58.1

Ingredients

Peanuts	¼ cup
Ginger	¼ inch
Sesame seeds	½ tbsp
Curry leaves	12 to 15
Oil	2 tsp
Salt	¼ tsp

Method

- Heat oil in a pan. Fry the peanuts on a low to medium flame for 3-4 minutes. Add the curry leaves and fry for a moment. Sauté for 2-3 minutes more on a low flame.
- Do not over-brown or burn this mixture, else the chutney may develop bitter tones.
- To make the chutney, add the contents in a grinder. Add ginger, sesame seeds and salt. Pour some water and grind the chutney to a smooth consistency. It can be made of thick or medium consistency. Check the salt and add more if required.

Healthy cooking tips

- Since peanuts are rich in fat, recipes using them require less oil.
- You can boil the sesame and then make a paste.

5. SEED-BASED CHUTNEY

KARELA CHUTNEY

A traditional Maharashtrian recipe prepared with bitter gourd, which makes for an ideal side dish during summers.

Skill level	Easy
Serving size	4
Place of origin	Maharashtra, India
Season most suited for consumption	Summer
Rich in nutrients	Calcium, Good Fats

Know your nutrition

Onion seeds: These are known to have anti-parasitic qualities and are effective in abscesses, orchitis, paralysis, facial palsy, migraine and amnesia-related problems. Its powder is effective in treating haemorrhoids and early stages of cataract. A solution of boiled seeds is very effective in calming inflammation as well as pain in the gums and teeth.

Sodium chloride: Sodium is an electrolyte that facilitates nerve impulses and regulates bodily functions such as heart rate, digestion, respiration, brain activity, and blood pressure. It helps to maintain the body's fluid balance.

Favourable for conditions

Infections, Constipation, Diabetes, Cardiac health, Bone health, PCOS, Pregnancy, Lactation

Calorie count

Serving Size	Energy (Kcal)	Carbohydrate (gm)	Protein (gm)	Fats (gm)	Calcium (mg)
1	246	8.6	8.1	19.8	178.8
4	983	34.2	32.2	79.4	715.4

Serving Size	Phosphorus (mg)	Iron (mg)	Total Fiber (mg)	Omega-3 (mg)	
1	100.1	5.9	5.7	24.1	
4	400.4	23.5	22.9	96.5	

Ingredients

Onion seeds	1 cup
Peanuts	¼ cup
Fresh coconut	¼ cup
Sesame seeds	2 tsp
Curry leaves	10-15
Salt	½ tsp

Method

- Roast onion seeds and sesame seeds separately in a pan on a low flame. Once the popping sound stops, remove the seeds from the flame and transfer them onto a plate and let them cool.
- In the same pan, dry roast fresh coconut, sesame seeds and curry leaves and let them cool.
- Then transfer all the ingredients in a mixer, and add salt to taste. Grind all ingredients into a coarse powder.
- Store in an air-tight container.

Healthy cooking tips

- Do not over-roast the onion seeds and sesame seeds as that can alter their properties.
- Coconut and peanut contain a good amount of oil, so while using them, use less additional oil in recipes.

SESAME SEEDS CHUTNEY

Maharashtrian chutney with a crunchy texture and a smoked flavour from til seeds, freshly grated coconut and aromatic spices.

Skill level	Easy
Serving	2
Place of origin	Maharashtra, India
Season most suited for consumption	Winter
Rich in nutrients	Calcium, Protein, Fiber

Know your nutrition

Black sesame seeds: Black sesame seeds are a good source of calcium, protein, manganese, iron, copper and phosphorous. They are rich in zinc and also a good source of concentrated calories. They can keep your bones strong and prevent osteoporosis. Sesame seeds also provide the body with vitamin E, which is required for a healthy skin. Black sesame seeds have a strong aroma and really good flavour. They are rich in fatty acids, minerals and dietary fiber.

Groundnut oil: It has vitamin E that protects from oxidative damage and reduces the risk of heart disease as well as cholesterol. It also maintains skin health. It is rich in omega-9 and omega-6 fatty acids and polyphenols like resveratrol that helps to maintain blood pressure, improves immune health, lowers Alzheimer's disease and prevents cancer.

Mustard seeds: It relieves flatulence, diarrhoea, parasite and worm infections, liver diseases, cardiovascular disorders, fevers, and also regulates immunity. It has antimicrobial, antiseptic and anti-inflammatory properties.

Favourable for conditions

Diabetes, Cardiac health, Bone health, PCOS, PMS, Pregnancy, Lactation, Skin disorders

Calorie count

Serving Size	Energy (Kcal)	Carbohydrate (gm)	Protein (gm)	Fats (gm)
1	138	5	3.6	11.3
2	276	9.9	7.2	22.7
Serving Size	Phosphorus (mg)	Total Fiber (mg)	Omega-3 (mg)	Calcium (mg)
1	45.4	3.6	47.8	144.7
2	90.9	7.2	95.5	289.4

Ingredients

Black sesame seeds	¼ cup
White urad dal (split)	1 tbsp
Fresh coconut, grated	¼ cup
Curry leaves	few
Salt	½ tsp
Groundnut Oil	1 tsp
Mustard seeds	½ tsp

Method

- Dry roast urad dal until brown. Stir in the black sesame seeds and fresh grated coconut. Roast for a few minutes.
- In a mixer grinder, add sesame seeds, urad dal and salt. Add some water. Grind it to a smooth, thick paste.
- Transfer the chutney to a serving bowl. In a tadka pan, heat oil on low flame and add mustard seeds. Allow the seeds to sputter. Immediately add curry leaves and allow to crackle for 5 seconds or more.

Healthy cooking tips

- Sesame seeds can be used widely. Just sprinkle these on your food or salad. One can prepare chikkis and chutney using the same process.

- Mustard seeds can be added in day-to-day recipes.
- Groundnut oil is a good source of MUFA so it is a healthier and more stable oil.
- Many people eat the curry leaf from dals and vegetables. Dry roast on a tawa and powder the curry leaves to add to any recipe.

🌿

TILKUT

A beneficial sesame seed chutney popular in Maharashtra, which is rich in many essential nutrients.

Skill level	Easy
Serving size	4
Place of origin	Maharashtra, India
Season most suited for consumption	Winter
Rich in nutrients	Calcium, Zinc, Protein, Good Fats

Know your nutrition

Dry coconut: Dried coconut carries many essential nutrients like dietary fiber, copper, manganese and selenium. It helps to improve brain function and also promotes a healthy brain. It even slows down the progress of any dreadful disease, like Alzheimer's, and helps in boosting the immune system. Dried coconut, which is packed with iron, can prevent anemia. It helps in preventing many digestive issues like constipation, duodenal ulcers and hemorrhoids as well.

Coriander seeds: These possess hypoglycaemic, hypolipidemic, antibacterial, antifungal, insecticidal and aflatoxin-controlling effects. They relieve flatulence, stimulate appetite and burn fat.

Favourable for conditions

Diabetes, Cardiac Health, Bone health, PCOS, Pregnancy, Lactation

Calorie count

Serving Size	Energy (Kcal)	Carbohydrate (gm)	Protein (gm)	Fats (gm)	Calcium (mg)
1	144	3.1	4.5	12.5	297.1
4	575	12.3	17.9	49.8	1188.3
Serving Size	Iron (mg)	Total Fiber (mg)	Omega-3 (mg)	Zinc (mg)	Phosphorus (mg)
1	3.6	4.3	29.5	1	72.1
4	14.4	17.3	118.2	3.9	288.5

Ingredients

Black sesame seeds	1 cup
Dry coconut	½ cup
Cumin seeds	1 tbsp
Coriander seeds	1 tbsp
Salt	½ tsp

Method

- Heat the pan and dry roast black sesame seeds, dry coconut, cumin seeds, and coriander seeds. Let the ingredients cool down.
- Now, grind coarsely and add salt according to the taste.
- Store the chutney in an air-tight container.

Healthy cooking tips

- Excess roasting can change the properties of black sesame seeds.
- You can add coconut powder instead of dry coconut as it contains less amount of fat.
- Ideally, coriander seeds should be ground fresh for each meal

to enhance their properties and to maximize the absorption of essential oils.

6. VEGETABLE-BASED CHUTNEY

AJWAIN LEAF CHUTNEY

A vibrant Indian chutney that has nutritious ingredients such as ajwain and curry leaves.

Skill level	Easy
Serving size	4
Place of origin	Haryana, Uttar Pradesh-India
Season most suited for consumption	Winter
Rich in nutrients	Good fats

Know your nutrition

Ajwain leaves are said to have a number of health benefits, including curing stomach problems, and improving appetite and digestion. They enhance the taste and flavour of everyday dishes, for everyday home remedies. Ajwain leaves can be boiled with water and made into a warm concoction to remedy persistent cold and cough.

Favourable for conditions

Digestion, Respiratory disorders, Diabetes, Cardiac Health, Lactation

Calorie count

Serving Size	Energy (Kcal)	Carbohydrate (gm)	Protein (gm)	Fats (gm)	Calcium (mg)	Phosphorus (mg)	Total Fiber (mg)	Omega-3 (mg)
1	32	1.5	1.6	1.9	46.1	16.4	2.1	47.4
4	128	6.1	6.5	7.4	184.6	65.7	8.5	189

Ingredients

Ajwain leaves	1 cup
Curry leaves	½ cup
Peanuts	¼ cup
Ginger	1 piece
Salt	½ tsp

Method

- First wash the ajwain and curry leaves. Grind in a mixer with peanuts and ginger.
- Add water to maintain consistency of chutney; then add salt in the chutney and grind it again to a fine paste.

Healthy cooking tips

- Wash the ajwain leaves. Dry them well and then use.
- Ginger is great for sea and motion sickness and nausea. It is used in detox drinks, raita, dal and curries.

BIRAKAI (RIDGE GOURD PEEL) CHUTNEY

A nourishing chutney enriched with the nutritive goodness of ridge gourd peel.

Skill level	Easy
Serving size	4
Place of origin	South India
Season most suited for consumption	All season
Rich in nutrients	Vitamin C, Zinc, Potassium, Iron, Beta-carotene

Know your nutrition

Ridge gourd: Ridge gourd is extremely rich in dietary fiber, vitamin-C, zinc, iron, riboflavin, magnesium and thiamine. It is low in saturated fat, cholesterol and calories that aid in weight loss. Ridge gourd contains a good amount of cellulose and is high in water content that helps to relieve constipation. It contains insulin-like peptides and alkaloids that help to reduce the sugar levels in blood and urine. It is high in beta-carotene, which is good for eyesight.

Tamarind: It is helpful in diarrhea, and has antibacterial properties due to the presence of lupeol. It also has anti-inflammatory and anti-nociceptive effects due to the presence of polyphenols and flavonoid, protects the liver and cures fluoride toxicity due to the presence of antioxidants.

Black gram: It is a plant-based source of protein, ideal for vegetarians and vegans. It is a source of zinc and potassium. It aids in digestion and prevents anemia. It improves heart health due to the presence of magnesium, fiber and potassium.

Favourable for conditions

Eye disorder, Diarrhea, Anemia, Heart disease

Calorie count

Serving Size	Energy (Kcal)	Carbohydrate (gm)	Protein (gm)	Fats (gm)	Calcium (mg)	Phosphorus (mg)	Total Fiber (mg)	Omega-3 (mg)
1	50	4.2	1.5	2.3	9.9	18.3	1.3	51.8
4	199	18.1	6	9.1	39.9	73.2	5.2	207.2

Ingredients

Chopped ridge gourd peel   1 cup
Urad dal   2 tbsp

Turmeric powder	¼ tsp
Mustard seeds	½ tsp
Tamarind	2 flakes
Oil	1 tbsp
Salt	1 tsp

Method

- Peel and chop the ridge gourd peel into small pieces. Heat oil. Add the urad dal and stir-fry till it is golden brown.
- Add the peels and stir-fry till the edges start to turn brown. Turn off the heat. Add salt, turmeric, and tamarind.
- Mix well and let it cool. Add a little water, and grind the fried ingredients to a smooth paste. Transfer it into a bowl.
- Heat 1 tsp oil. Add the mustard seeds and wait till they crackle.
- Add the tempering and mix well. Serve the chutney with rice, idli or dosa.

Healthy cooking tips

- Instead of discarding the peel, you can use it to make this chutney.
- Soak the tamarind in the water for 1 hour before adding it to the grinder.
- Mustard seeds have antimicrobial properties and help improve immunity. They are advised to be incorporated into day-to-day recipes.

COCONUT-CARROT CHUTNEY

A combination of sweetness from coconut and sourness from green mango.

| Skill level | Easy |
| Serving size | 4 |

Place of origin	Maharashtra, India
Season most suited for consumption	Summer
Rich in nutrients	Beta-carotene, Sodium, Potassium, MCTs

Know your nutrition

Coconut: Coconut is low in carbohydrates and high in fiber, which helps stabilize blood sugar. It also has an anti-diabetic effect due to its arginine content. It is high in antioxidants, which also prevent oxidative damage. It also has a beneficial effect on heart health and is also good for skin and hair health.

Carrot: It is a good source of vitamins A, B6 and K, biotin, and potassium. It improves eyesight and immune function, provides satiety and prevents constipation. It also reduces the risk of cancer.

Raw Mango: Raw mango boosts your metabolism, thus helping you burn more calories, and prevents dehydration. It is also high in niacin, which helps boost cardiovascular health. It is rich in antioxidants such as vitamins A, C and E, folate and fiber. Thus, it boosts immunity and improves digestive health. It also has a good amount of pectin, so it can prevent cancer and cholesterol. It is a good source of energy.

Favourable for conditions

Vitamin A Deficiencies, Eye disorders, Anemia, Pregnancy, Diabetes, Bone health

Calorie count

Serving Size	Energy (Kcal)	Carbohydrate (gm)	Total Fiber (mg)	Protein (gm)	Fats (gm)
1	97	3.6	2.5	1.7	7.6
4	389	14.4	10.3	6.8	30.4

Serving Size	Omega-3 (mg)	Beta-carotene (mcg)	Sodium (mg)	Potassium (mg)	
1	13.1	560	230.4	101.2	
4	52.5	2240.1	921.7	404.9	

Ingredients

Coconut	50 gms
Carrot	1 small
Green Mango	½ of a medium-sized fruit
Curd	2 tbsp
Curry Leaves	3-4 leaves
Coriander Leaves	3-4 sprigs
Mustard Seeds	¼ tsp
Crushed Peanuts	1 tbsp
Oil	1 tsp
Salt	¼ tsp

Method

- Take coconut, grated carrot, green mango and coriander leaves in a blender. Add curd, salt, and sugar to it and blend it once. Do not blend much as we need it to be of a thick consistency.
- Take a small vessel for the vaghar and put oil, mustard seeds, crushed peanuts, and curry leaves in it. Heat it and put on the blended chutney.
- Mix it thoroughly and serve with thalipith or any parathas.

Healthy cooking tips

- Wash the carrots well; do not peel them.
- Cooking carrots enhances the lycopene content and increases vitamin A availability.
- Raw mangoes are used to prepare chutneys and pickles, or can be added to dals or pulavs.
- Coconut can be used in water, milk, or grated form in curries and gravies.

- Coconut itself contains a good amount of oil so while using coconut, use less oil in the recipe.

❧

CURRY LEAVES CHUTNEY

Delicious Indian curry leaves recipe, which has many beneficial qualities.

Skill level	Easy
Serving	2
Place of origin	Assam, Telangana
Season most suited for consumption	All season
Rich in nutrients	Vitamin C, Fiber, Iron

Know your nutrition

Curry leaves: Curry leaves promote gastrointestinal health, prevent diarrhea and diabetes, reduce cholesterol since they contain a good amount of fiber and anti-diabetic properties, and prevent cancer as they are rich in antioxidants such as vitamin C. They are rich in iron, which helps in increasing hemoglobin. The leaves are beneficial for women who suffer from calcium deficiency, osteoporosis, etc.

Coconut: Coconuts are low in carbohydrates and high in fiber which helps stabilize blood sugar. They are antidiabetic due to arginine. They are high in antioxidants, which also prevent oxidative damage. They are also beneficial for heart health and good for the skin as well as hair.

Favourable for conditions

Diabetes, Cardiac health, Bone health, PCOS, Pregnancy, Lactation, Skin and hair disorders

Calorie count

Serving Size	Energy (Kcal)	Carbohydrate (gm)	Protein (gm)	Fats (gm)	Calcium (mg)
1	54	0.6	0.4	5.6	7.8
2	107	1.2	0.9	11.1	15.5
Serving Size	Total Fiber (mg)	Omega-3 (mg)	Sodium (mg)	Vitamin C (mg)	Phosphorus (mg)
1	1	20	216.6	0.1	4.9
2	2.1	40.1	433.2	0.2	9.9

Ingredients

Curry leaves	1 cup
Grated coconut	1 tbsp
Salt	¼ tsp
Oil	1 tsp
Mustard seeds	¾ tsp

Method

- Wash the curry leaves and drain the water. Pat dry.
- Heat oil in pan, add mustard seeds, curry leaves, and sauté on low flame for 2-3 minutes. Add grated coconut and sauté for a few more seconds.
- Switch off the flame, add salt and allow it to cool. Grind the mixture and add some water to make a smooth paste. Consistency should neither be thick nor thin, so add water accordingly.

Healthy cooking tips

- Curry leaves are a versatile vegetable and a great flavouring agent. They contain a good amount of fiber and anti-diabetic properties.
- Coconut contains a good amount of oil so while using coconut, use less oil in the recipes.

DIL-YOGURT DIP

A flavoursome yogurt dip with a good worth of bright fresh dill leaves.

Skill level	Easy
Serving size	1
Place of origin	India
Season most suited for consumption	Monsoon
Rich in nutrients	Calcium, Vitamins A and C

Know your nutrition

Curd: Curd is rich in lactoccus lactis which encourages the growth of healthy gut flora and promotes digestion. It also improves muscles since it is rich in calcium and is a good probiotic food that keeps the ecosystem balanced. It prevents the activity of harmful microorganisms. The bioactive protein in curd also reduces blood pressure and cholesterol levels.

Dill leaves: Fresh dill is very low in calories, yet a good source of vitamin C that helps in boosting immunity, bone health and vitamin A, which improves eye sight. It is a good source of manganese that supports normal functioning of your brain, nervous system, and metabolism. It is a moderate source of calcium, copper, magnesium, potassium, riboflavin, and zinc. It also contains antioxidants like flavonoids, terpenoids and tannins, which help in reducing inflammation, heart disease, Alzheimer's, rheumatoid arthritis, and certain forms of cancer.

Favourable for conditions

Digestion, Probiotic, Anemia, Diabetes, Cardiac health, Bone health, PCOS, Children

Calorie count

Serving Size	Energy (Kcal)	Carbohydrate (gm)	Protein (gm)	Fats (gm)	Calcium (mg)
1	83	5.9	4.9	4.8	143
Serving Size	Iron (mg)	Folate (mcg)	Beta carotene (mcg)	Vitamin C (mg)	Phosphorus (mg)
1	1.1	25.8	715.5	5.7	66.9

Ingredients

Curd	2 cups
Dill leaves	For garnish
Salt	¼ tsp

Method

- Spread curd on a muslin cloth and get the ends together.
- Make a knot and hang it just above the kitchen sink.
- Place a colander or filter over a container to gather whey.
- Leave it for about 30 minutes and then squeeze out the whey.
- Put the cloth on the colander and cover it.
- Keep it in the refrigerator for about 4 hours.
- Add fresh dill leaves and salt. Serve chilled.

Healthy cooking tips

- During cold weather, curd takes a longer time to set, and doesn't get sour for a long time.

❀

MORINGA LEAVES CHUTNEY PODI

Scrumptuous South Indian chutney recipe, which offers freshness from drumstick leaves.

Skill level	Easy
Serving size	1
Place of origin	South India
Season most suited for consumption	All season
Rich in nutrients	Vitamins A (beta carotene), Calcium, Phosphorus, Omega 3

Know your nutrition:

Moringa leaves: They reduce inflammation, are high in antioxidant power since they are rich in vitamin C, quercetin and chlorogenic acid which fight infections. Moringa leaves help in treating cancer since they are rich in niazimicin (an anti-cancer agent) that restrains the development of cancer cells. The leaves improve heart health by effectively reducing cholesterol levels, and improve bone health as they are rich in calcium and phosphorous, which increase bone mass and structural strength.

Peanuts: Peanuts are high in energy. They improve heart health and prevent gallstones. They contain niacin, which protects against Alzheimer's disease and cognitive decline. Peanuts are a rich source of folate, which is good for pregnant women. The magnesium content of peanuts helps to reduce inflammation.

Favourable for conditions

Weight loss, Diabetes, Anemia, Cardiac Health, Bone health, PCOS, Pregnancy, Lactation

Calorie count

Serving Size	Energy (Kcal)	Carbohydrate (gm)	Protein (gm)	Fats (gm)	Calcium (mg)
1	76	3.8	3	4.38	41.11

Serving Size	Phosphorus (mg)	Total Fiber (mg)	Omega-3 (mg)	Beta carotene (mcg)	
1	39.31	2.81	63.15	1670.5	

Ingredients

Moringa Leaves (the fresher the better) 1 cup

Peanuts	1 tbsp
Black Pepper Powder	¼ tsp
Methi Seeds	1/3 tsp
Cumin Seeds	1/3 tsp
Salt	¼ tsp

Method

- Heat oil in a pan on medium heat; roast the peanut, black pepper, fenugreek seeds, and cumin seeds.
- Once well roasted, stir in the Moringa leaves and sauté for a few seconds till leaves are crisp and dry.
- Cool the chutney mixture completely and grind it into a coarse powder in the food processor along with some salt.
- Serve along with hot steamed rice.

Healthy cooking tips

- Moringa is a versatile plant and a great flavouring agent.
- It contains a good amount of fiber and has anti-diabetic properties.
- Many people discard drumstick leaves from dals and vegetables. Dry roast on a tawa and powder the curry leaves to add to recipes. Can be added to smoothies and salads as well.

❧

RADISH CHUTNEY

A yummy chutney prepared with radishes.

Skill level	Moderate
Serving size	2
Place of origin	Assam, Tamil Nadu

Season most suited for consumption   Winter
Rich in nutrients   Protein, Good fats, Vitamin A, Vitamin C.

Know your nutrition

Radish: High in vitamins A, E, C, B6 and K. Also, high on antioxidants, fiber, zinc, potassium, phosphorus, magnesium, copper, calcium, iron and manganese. It controls blood pressure. Aids in acidity, obesity, gastric problems and nausea. Good for skin and hydration and also controls the damage of RBCs.

Black gram: It is a plant-based source of protein, ideal for vegetarians and vegans. It is a source of zinc and potassium. It aids in digestion and prevents anemia. It improves heart health due to the presence of magnesium, fibre and potassium.

Fenugreek seeds: Fenugreek seeds, also known as methi seeds, are a good source of dietary fiber, which is a very important nutrient in controlling cholesterol and other toxins. The mineral component present in the seeds like iron, zinc, calcium, selenium, etc., provides essential control on body fluids, blood pressure and heart rate.

Favourable for conditions

Diabetes, Cardiac health, Monsoons, Athletes

Calorie count

Serving Size	Energy (Kcal)	Carbohydrate (gm)	Protein (gm)	Fats (gm)	Calcium (mg)
1	131	6.9	2.1	10.1	21.1
2	261	13.9	4.1	20.1	42.1
Serving Size	Total Fiber (mg)	Beta carotene (mcg)	Omega-3 (mg)	Vitamin C (mg)	Phosphorus (mg)
1	3.3	70.5	96.6	1.8	30.6
2	6.7	141	193.3	3.6	61.2

Ingredients

Radish, grated	1 cup
Black Urad Dal (Split)	2 tsps
Fresh Coconut	¼ cup
Turmeric Powder	¼ tsp
Salt	¼ tsp
Sesame (Gingelly) Oil	2 tsps
Black Urad Dal (Split)	1 tsp
Mustard Seeds	1 tsp
Curry Leaves	¼ cup
Methi Seeds	¼ tsp

Method

- Warm a pan over medium heat. Add urad dal and roast. Once it turns light golden brown, add the grated radish, salt, coconut and turmeric powder.
- Sauté until the radish is softened. Add the cooked radish chutney ingredients into a turbo chop and make a smooth paste.
- Add 2 tsp of water, if required, while grinding. Once done, transfer to a serving bowl.
- For the tadka, heat oil over medium heat; add mustard seeds, methi seeds and urad dal and allow the dal to roast and turn golden brown. Stir in the curry leaves and pour the tadka over the radish chutney.

Healthy cooking tips

- Wash the radish well and use it. People suffering from bloating should avoid eating radish.
- Coconut itself contains a good amount of oil so while using coconut, use less oil in recipes.
- Sprouted fenugreek seeds can be used for better health benefits.
- Consume urad dal only in the afternoon. It can be used as a

part of tempering in a lot of dals and chutneys because it gives a nice crunch and increases the protein content.

✤

RAISIN-TOMATO CHUTNEY

Homemade finger-licking chutney with a combination of tomatoes, black raisins and sesame seeds.

Skill level	Easy
Serving size	2
Place of origin	Maharashtra, India
Season most suited for consumption	All season
Rich in nutrients	Vitamin A, Protein, Dietary Fiber

Know your nutrition

Tomatoes: Tomatoes are a good source of several vitamins and minerals such as vitamins C, K and B9, and potassium. They also have a high content of lycopene and beta-carotene that reduces the risk of cancer, heart diseases and neuro-degenerative diseases. They are a rich in dietary fiber that provide satiety. They also protect the skin and promote eye health.

Grapes: Grapes are rich in antioxidants. Resveratrol prevents cardiovascular diseases, improves learning, memory and mood, lowers blood sugar and age-related macular degeneration, reduces inflammation and protects against the development of cancer. They improves the lipid profile and cures urinary tract infections as well.

Sesame oil: It contains sesamol and sesaminol, two antioxidants that help to reduce cell damage by free radicals and protect against oxidative damage. It helps to reduce inflammation and prevents arthritis. It is rich in omega-6 fatty acids that help to prevent heart disease and cancer and reduce cholesterol. It regulates blood sugar levels. It contains collagen that helps to heal wounds and burns. It also improves hair health and provides relief from other joint pains.

Favourable for conditions

Pregnancy, Children, Cardiac health, Infections, Athletes

Calorie count

Serving Size	Energy (Kcal)	Carbohydrate (gm)	Protein (gm)	Fats (gm)	Calcium (mg)
1	192	19.6	0.8	9.6	25.2
2	385	39.1	1.5	19.3	50.4
Serving Size	Phosphorus (mg)	Total Fiber (mg)	Omega-3 (mg)	B-carotene (mcg)	
1	40.4	5.8	39	1,414.5	
2	80.8	11.5	78	2,829	

Ingredients

Tomatoes, roughly chopped	4
Turmeric powder	¼ tsp
Groundnut oil	1 tsp
Salt	¼ tsp
Sesame (Gingelly) oil	1 tsp
Black raisins	2 tsp
Sesame seeds	½ tsp
Curry leaves	4

Method

- Heat oil in a small pan, add the chopped tomatoes, salt and turmeric powder. Sauté until the tomatoes are nice and soft and almost all the water has evaporated.
- Allow the mixture to cool and then grind into a smooth paste.

- Heat oil in another small pan; add mustard seeds, curry leaves and sesame seeds, and allow them to crackle.
- Pour this seasoning over the ground tomato chutney, give it a good stir and add black raisins on top.

Healthy cooking tips

- People with elevated uric acid can scoop out or remove the seeds in tomatoes and then eat.
- Sesame seeds can be sprinkled on food or chutney.
- Sesame oil is used as a traditional cooking oil to enhance the flavour of many cuisines, and also has a nutty aroma and taste.

RED PEPPER DIP

A lip-smacking red pepper dip recipe that blends exotic flavours and can be served with a mezze platter.

Skill level	Easy
Serving size	1
Place of origin	India
Season most suited for consumption	All season
Rich in nutrients	Vitamins A and C

Know your nutrition

Bell peppers: Bell peppers provide key antioxidants such as lycopene, beta carotene, lutein and zeaxanthin, which protect the body from free radicals, and help reduce the risk of cancer, heart disease and neuro-degenerative disease. They are rich in vitamins A and C, as well as a moderate source for vitamins E and K. Manganese and potassium are also found in bell peppers. They also have high amounts of fiber, which provides fullness to the stomach and decreases digestion-related problems. They also protect the eyesight and promote bone health.

Rock salt: Rock salt contains various trace minerals like manganese, iron, copper and zinc, which is known to improve digestion and is a natural way to relieve stomach pain. Mineral baths are a great way to relieve sore or cramped muscles.

Favourable for conditions

Infection, Anemia, Diabetes, Cardiac health, PCOS

Calorie count

Serving Size	Energy (Kcal)	Carbohydrate (gm)	Protein (gm)	Fats (gm)	Calcium (mg)
1	225	13.7	1.6	10.7	47.4
Serving Size	Total Fiber (mg)	Phosphorus (mg)	Vitamin A (mcg)	Vitamin C (mg)	Omega-3 (mg)
1	8.7	67.7	518.4	49.7	236.2

Ingredients

Red bell pepper, chopped into 1 inch pieces	1
Tomatoes, sliced	2 large
Cumin	1 tsp
Coriander leaves	2 tbsp
Sendha salt	¼ tsp
Cooking oil	1 tbsp

For tempering/tadka:

Oil	1 tsp
Mustard Seeds	½ tsp
Curry Leaves	A sprig
Asafoetida	1 pinch

Method

- Heat 1.5 tsps of oil in a vessel. Once the oil is hot, reduce the flame, add chana dal, cumin and red chilies and sauté till the dal turns brown. Add coriander leaves and sauté for 2 min. Remove the contents from the vessel and keep aside to cool.

- In the same vessel, add one tbsp of oil, add three bell pepper pieces and sauté for 6 min. Add the tomatoes and sauté for 9-10 min on low to medium flame. Turn off heat and cool.

- Blend the dal mixture till coarse. Then add the cooled ingredients (tomatoes and red bell peppers) in conjunction with the salt and grind to a fine paste. Remove in a serving bowl.

- Heat one tsp of oil in a small pan, add the mustard seeds and allow them to sputter. Add the curry leaves and asafoetida and turn off the heat.

- Pour this tempering over the chutney and serve with appams.

Healthy cooking tips

- Red and yellow bell peppers can be substituted with capsicum.

❧

RIDGE GOURD PEEL CHUTNEY

Authentic Andhra Pradesh chutney recipe that is infused with the aromatic native flavours from spices, grated coconut and nutritive ridge gourd peel.

Skill level	Moderate
Serving size	3
Place of origin	Andhra Pradesh, India
Season most suited for consumption	Summer, Monsoon
Rich in nutrients	Dietary Fiber, Vitamin C, Magnesium

Know your nutrition

Ridge gourd: Ridge gourd is extremely rich in dietary fiber and enriched with all the vital elements that include vitamin C, zinc, iron, riboflavin, magnesium, and thiamine. It is low in saturated fat, cholesterol and calories, which aids in weight loss. Ridge gourd contains a good amount of cellulose and is high in water content that helps to relieve constipation. It contains insulin-like peptides and alkaloids, which helps to reduce sugar levels in the blood and urine. It is high in beta-carotene, which is good for enhancing the eyesight.

Peppercorn: Pepper is an important antioxidant, which helps in cognitive brain functioning. It is an antidepressant that boosts nutrient absorption and improves gastrointestinal functionality. Its free radical-scavenging activity might help control the progression of tumour growth. Charak Samhita states its uses in curing abdominal disorders.

Cumin seeds: Ayurveda proves the benefits of cumin in the gastrointestinal, reproductive, nervous and immune system. It has antioxidant, antimicrobial and chemoprotective properties. Many other remarkable health benefits include anti-diabetic, antiseptic, relief from flatulence and metabolism stimulation.

Favourable for conditions

Diabetes, Cardiac health, Bone health, PCOS

Calorie count

Serving Size	Energy (Kcal)	Carbohydrate (gm)	Protein (gm)	Fats (gm)	Calcium (mg)
1	150	1.7	0.7	12.1	8.1
3	450	5	2.2	36.5	24.3
Serving Size	Total Fiber (mg)	Phosphorus (mg)	Vitamin C (mg)	Magnesium (mg)	Omega-3 (mg)
1	2	13	0.4	5.4	25.7
3	6	39.1	1.1	16.2	77.2

Ingredients

Ridge gourd with peels	¾ cup
Grated coconut	½ cup
Peppercorns	½ tsp
Cumin seeds	½ tsp
Oil	1 tbsp
Salt	½ tsp
Ghee/Oil	1 tbsp
Mustard seeds	½ tsp
Curry leaves	2 leaflets

Method

- Remove the hard, sharp ridges off the peel using a knife. The whole peel may be used in the chutney.
- Roughly chop the ridge gourd peels and keep it aside. You can add the gourd's inner flesh too, but it makes the chutney a little mushy unlike the dry chutney you get with just the peels.
- Heat oil in a kadhai and add the cumin seeds. When they start popping, add peppercorns and let them sizzle for a few seconds.
- Now add the roughly chopped ridge gourd peels, salt and ½ cup of water. Cook them until the peels are cooked through with a closed lid.
- Once the peels are completely cooked, remove them and let them cool completely.
- Once cooled, grind all the ingredients in the wok with grated coconut into a coarse or smooth paste using as little water as possible. The chutney is usually served dry.
- Transfer the ground chutney into a bowl. Check and adjust salt. Season the chutney if you wish. Chutney tastes great even without the seasoning.
- Seasoning: Heat oil/ghee in a tempering pan, and add the mustard seeds. When they start popping, add the curry leaves and let them sizzle. Add this seasoning to the chutney and blend well.

Healthy cooking tips

- Ridge gourd is used in making salads and juices. It is a healthy vegetable widely used for weight loss. It is low in calories and can be cooked in minimal oil. The peels can be used to make chutney, causing zero waste.
- Coconut itself contains a good amount of oil so while using coconut, use less oil in the recipes.
- Black pepper can be added with turmeric for better absorption and together they help to burn fat.

WHEATGRASS CHUTNEY

A wholesome chutney that incorporates freshly blended green leaves.

Skill level	Easy
Serving size	3
Place of origin	India
Season most suited for consumption	Winter
Rich in nutrients	Vitamin C, Good fats.

Know your nutrition

Wheatgrass: It is thought to be antioxidant and anti-inflammatory, which can help to stimulate the immune system, detoxify the body and help the digestive system by getting rid of harmful bacteria. The high amount of chlorophyll (the substance that gives plants their green colour) in the young grass, is useful in the improvement of red blood cell count. It is also said to help in balancing blood sugar and cholesterol.

Lemon: Lemon has vitamin C. Sprinkling some over iron-rich foods would aid in better absorption of iron from the source.

It has anti-viral and anti-inflammatory properties and helps in boosting immunity, and lowers the risk of heart diseases like atherosclerosis, diabetes, cancers, and kidney stones.

Favourable for conditions

Anemia, Infection, Diabetes, Cardiac health, Bone health, PCOS, Pregnancy

Calorie count

Serving Size	Energy (Kcal)	Carbohydrate (gm)	Protein (gm)	Fats (gm)	Calcium (mg)
1	230	15.4	11	15.5	67.7
3	547	42.2	26.9	34.2	184.8
Serving Size	Iron (mg)	Total Fiber (mg)	Omega-3 (mg)	Vitamin C (mg)	Phosphorus (mg)
1	6.8	5.2	78.9	34.8	56.9
3	19.2	13.6	236.7	104.3	123.6

Ingredients

Fresh wheatgrass	25 gm
Coriander	25 gm
Mint	50 gm
Ginger	10 gm
Lime	1
Peanut	25 gm
Coconut	25 gm
Salt	½ tsp

Method

- Grind all ingredients to a fine paste.
- Pour into a clean bowl.
- Add salt and lemon, and mix well.

Best served with

- Lunch or dinner
- Roti or thepla
- Dhokla, idli, or appam

Healthy cooking tips

- Add tomato, cucumber, cabbage and make a veggie wrap.
- Lime can be added with wheatgrass to boost vitamin C intake. Wheatgrass can be mixed with pudina, coriander, or coconut for better health effects.
- Use small spoons for measuring to consciously reduce the quantity of salt consumed daily.

❧

YELLOW PUMPKIN WITH VEGETABLE PEEL CHUTNEY

A wholesome Andhra-style appetizing chutney of pumpkin, highly nutritious vegetable peels and seeds.

Skill level	Moderate
Serving size	2
Place of origin	Andhra Pradesh, India
Season most suited for consumption	All season
Rich in nutrients	Magnesium, Iron, Fiber

Know your nutrition

Pumpkin: Pumpkin has antioxidant content such beta carotene that protects the body from free radicals. It is also rich in vitamin A that helps in improving eyesight and is a good source of vitamins C and E, iron, potassium and folate. It has high content of water and also has high amounts of fiber that provides satiety and decreases digestion-related problems. Augments immunity and promotes eye health.

Pumpkin seeds: Antioxidants in pumpkin seeds reduce the risk of cancer, fight infection and reduce inflammation. They improve prostate and bladder health. High content of magnesium helps to lower blood pressure and reduce the risk of heart disease. Magnesium also helps to control blood sugar levels. Pumpkin seed contains tryptophan, which helps to improve sleep. High fiber content in seeds helps to prevent constipation.

Watermelon seeds: Watermelon seeds are a good source of iron, which helps to prevent anemia. The calcium content promotes bone health. Manganese, protein and copper in the seeds are good for hair and skin health.

Favourable for conditions

Diabetes, Cardiac health, Bone health, PCOS, Pregnancy, lactation

Calorie count

Serving Size	Energy (Kcal)	Carbohydrate (gm)	Protein (gm)	Fats (gm)	Calcium (mg)
1	153	15.6	2.5	4.2	26.9
2	306	31.1	5	8.4	53.7
Serving Size	Phosphorus (mg)	Total Fiber (mg)	Omega-3 (mg)	Magnesium (mg)	
1	67.8	11.5	124.5	36.5	
2	135.6	22.9	249.1	53	

Ingredients

Two cups of vegetable peels (white and yellow pumpkins, bottle gourd and snake gourd) thoroughly washed and chopped

Pumpkin	1 inch piece
Mustard	½ tsp
Ginger	1-inch piece
Coriander, chopped	A handful
Salt	¼ tsp

Oil for sautéing	1 tsp
Curry leaves	4-5 leaves
Watermelon seeds	1 tbsp
Pumpkin seeds	1 tbsp

Method

- Heat oil in a kadhai. Add mustard seeds, and curry leaves, and sauté a little.
- Add the chopped peels and pieces of pumpkin. Add a pinch of salt to speed up the cooking. Sauté well till the raw smell goes away and the pumpkin is cooked. Take care not to burn the peel. Add a little water to it.
- Add the peels and a piece of ginger in the mixer and grind. Halfway through, add the coriander leaves. The chutney has to be a bit coarse and not super-fine. Add the pumpkin and watermelon seeds on top.

Healthy cooking tips

- Pumpkin is used as a thickening agent. It can be used as an alternative to potato as well.
- Ginger is great to reduce motion sickness and nausea. It is used in detox drinks, raita, dal and curries.
- Pumpkin seeds can be eaten as a snack. They have a very high magnesium content so they can be used as a sleep inducer.
- As a low-cost alternative to cashew nuts, people often add watermelon seed powder to thicken a gravy.

7. INTERNATIONAL CHUTNEY

HOMESTYLE JAIN SALSA

A homemade salsa dip that offers exotic intercontinental flavours.

| Skill level | Easy |

Serving size	1
Place of origin	Spain, Europe
Season most suited for consumption	All season
Rich in nutrients	Vitamins A and C

Know your nutrition

Honey: Honey is composed of fructose and glucose sugars. It also contains traces of enzymes, amino acids, vitamins B and C, minerals and antioxidants. It has antimicrobial properties and treats digestive issues.

Oregano: Oregano is rich in antioxidants, which are compounds that help fight damage from harmful free radicals. It also reduces inflammation and the risk of heart disease, diabetes and autoimmune conditions.

Favourable for conditions

Diabetes, Cardiac health, Cancer prevention, PCOS, Pregnancy, lactation

Calorie count

Serving Size	Energy (Kcal)	Carbohydrate (gm)	Protein (gm)	Fats (gm)	Calcium (mg)
1	234	26.7	1.1	8.8	40.4
Serving Size	Total Fiber (mg)	Phosphorus (mg)	Vitamin A (mcg)	Vitamin C (mg)	Omega-3 (mg)
1	10.3	59.8	785	47.9	77.5

Ingredients

Tomatoes	6
Capsicum, finely chopped	¼ cup
Cumin Powder	1 tsp
Oregano	1.5 tsp

Coriander Leaves	1 tbsp
Oil	1 tbsp
Honey	1 tsp
Amchoor	1 tsp

Method

- Cut tomatoes into halves and put them in boiling water. Then remove the skin of the tomatoes.
- Heat oil in a kadhai and sauté the capsicum.
- Cut the tomatoes in very small pieces and add to the oil.
- Add oregano, salt, honey and jeera powder, and cook for 5 minutes on slow flame.
- Garnish with honey and coriander leaves.

Healthy cooking tips

- Tomatoes can be blanched. Individuals with elevated uric acid problems can scoop out or remove the seeds before eating tomatoes.
- Coriander is a versatile vegetable used in making chutney and garnishing dishes.

5

DECODING FOOD: THE VEDIC WAY

*'It is every man's right to be independent;
but it is every man's duty to be interdependent.'*

—Mahatma Gandhi

SHADARASAS: The Six Tastes and their Effect on our Body

INTRODUCTION TO SHADRASA

Shadrasa is derived from the Sanskrit word 'shad', which means six types, while the word 'rasa' means taste perception, which is felt through the 'rasanendriya' i.e., tongue.

As per modern science, the taste organ is nothing but the taste buds. Each taste bud is made up of 100-150 receptors. The life of each receptor is one to two weeks after which these receptors are replaced by another. As per Ayurveda, there are six types of rasas (shadrasa):

- Madhura (sweet),
- Amla (sour)
- Lavana (salty)
- Katu (pungent)
- Tikta (bitter)
- Kashya (astringent)

TASTE MAHABHUTA RELATION

The basic five elements can be related to dietary foods:

- Ether/space for popcorn/wafers, etc.
- Air for beans/cabbage/cookies, etc.
- Fire for chilies/pepper/ginger, etc.
- Water for soups/melons, etc.
- Earth for fried foods/cheese, etc.

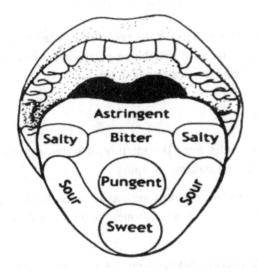

The basic principle of the diet is that physical changes as well as mental effects are often observed after the consumption of various foods. In this way, food can, directly and indirectly, affect the three doshas of an individual. The Panchamahabhuta, which are non-living entities, combine by permutation gives rise to Tridoshas. These Tridoshas have some basic chemical structures which further give rise to the dominant rasa.

EVOLUTION OF TASTE

Taste	Evolution	Doshas
Madhura rasa	Prithvi and Ap (earth+water)	
Amla rasa	Prithvi and Agni (earth+fire)	
Lavana rasa	Ap and Agni (water+fire)	Kaphadosha
Katu rasa	Vayu and Agni (air+fire)	Pitta dosha
Tikta rasa	Vayu and Akasha (air+ether)	Vatadosha
Kashaya rasa	Vayu and Prithvi (air+earth)	

ANURASA: The Anurasa is the secondary taste perception after primary taste. The Rasa is stable in a dry state, whereas Anurasa is unstable. E.g.: Honey astringent sub-taste.

1. MADHURA

Sweet taste results from the mixture of water and earth and is heavy, moist, and naturally cooling.

Benefits of moderate consumption: It promotes the growth of plasma, blood, fat, muscles, bones, marrow, and reproductive fluids.

Risk due to excess consumption: Excess consumption of sweet foods aggravates kapha dosa, which results in obesity, risk of cardiovascular disorders, stroke, development of kidney stones, softening of tissues, lethargy, hypersomnia, increase in cholesterol levels, impairment of digestive process, dystrophy of the tissues in the mouth and throat, and discomfort in urinating.

Source: Foods with sweet taste include sugar, honey, maple syrup, dates, rice, wheat, milk, milk products, most grains (especially wheat, rice, and barley), many legumes (like beans and lentils), sweet fruits (such as bananas and mangoes, dates, etc.), and certain cooked vegetables (such as carrots, sweet potatoes, and beets).

2. AMLA

Sour taste consists of earth and fire and is hot, light, and moist, naturally.

Benefits of moderate consumption: In moderation, sour foods are refreshing. They pacify vata but increase pitta and kapha. They stimulate the appetite, improve digestion, energize the body, nourish the heart, relieve thirst, maintain acidity, sharpen the senses, and help extract minerals such as iron from food. They also nourish all the vital tissues (dhatus).

Risk due to excess consumption: Excess consumption can cause hyperacidity, ulcers, and perforations. Its fermenting action can be toxic to the blood and cause skin conditions like acne, dermatitis, eczema, psoriasis, boils, and edema, as well as burning sensations in the throat, chest, heart, bladder and urinary tract.

Source: All citrus fruits like amla, lime and lemon, and other food products include unripe mangoes, green grapes, sour cream, yogurt, vinegar and fermented foods.

3. LAVANA

Salty taste consists of fire and water and is hot, heavy, and moist, naturally.

Benefits of moderate consumption: In moderation, salty taste improves the flavour of food, stimulates salivation, improves digestion and absorption, lubricates tissues, liquefies mucous, maintains mineral balance, aids in the elimination of wastes, balances blood pressure by maintaining electrolytes and calms the nerves. Due to its tendency to draw in water, it also improves the radiance of the skin and promotes overall growth within the body.

Risk due to excess consumption: Excess consumption of salt in the diet makes the blood viscous and thick, can cause hypertension, and aggravates skin conditions. Heat sensations, fainting, wrinkling, and baldness could also be because of excess salt, as well as edema, water retention, ulcers, bleeding disorders, skin eruptions, hyperacidity, and hypertension. It also increases pitta dosha leading to hyperacidity.

Source: Sea salt, rock salt and table salt, sea vegetables (like seaweed and kelp), and salted chips, nuts and pickles are some of the sources of salty taste.

4. KATU

Pungent taste derives from the elements of fire and air and is hot, dry and light.

Benefits of moderate consumption: Pungent taste stimulates digestion, clears the sinuses, promotes sweating and detoxification, dispels gas, aids circulation, improves metabolism, breaks up clots, kills parasites and germs, and relieves muscle pain.

Risk due to excess consumption: Excess consumption irritates, can cause choking, fainting, fainting fits, and fatigue. If it leads to a pitta aggravation, it can cause diarrhea, heartburn, nausea, peptic ulcers, colitis, and skin conditions. If it provokes vata, it can cause tremors, insomnia, and muscle pain.

Source: Chili pepper, cayenne pepper, habanera pepper, black pepper, clove and asafoetida are sources of this taste. Apart from this, spices such as cinnamon, basil, mint, thyme, mustard, ginger, garlic, and onion are also pungent in taste.

5. TIKTA

The bitter taste consists of air and ether and is light, cooling, and dry, naturally.

Benefits of moderate consumption: Bitter taste is a powerful detoxifying agent, and has antibiotic, antiparasitic, and antiseptic qualities. It's also helpful in reducing weight, water retention, skin rashes, fever, burning sensations, and nausea. Bitter helps to alleviate burning sensations, itching, fainting, and obstinate skin disorders. It reduces fever and stimulates the firmness of skin and muscles. In small doses, it can relieve intestinal gas and work as a digestive tonic.

Risk due to excess consumption: Excess consumption of bitter taste may deplete plasma, blood, muscles, fat, bone marrow, and semen, which can lead to sexual debility. It also causes the loss of cheerfulness of the mind, delusion fainting, dryness of the mouth, and increases vata dosha.

Source: Sources of this taste are green leafy vegetables such as spinach, neem and kale; creeper vegetables like zucchini, bitter gourd and eggplant; herbs and spices like turmeric, fenugreek, dandelion root, and aloe vera; coffee; tea; and certain fruits such as grapefruits, olives, and bitter melon.

6. KASHAYA

Astringent taste results from the mixture of air and earth and is dry, cooling, and naturally heavy.

Benefits of moderate consumption: Its qualities are cooling, drying, and heavy. Moderately, it aids in healing ulcers and promotes clotting.

Risk due to excess consumption: In excess, it may cause constipation, distension of abdomen, heart spasm, and stagnant circulation. It may also result in the depletion of sperm and affect the sexual drive. It may give rise to a range of neuromuscular disorders.

It also provokes the disturbances of vata, causes pericardial pain, thirst, obstruction of the channels of circulation of fluids, faecal retention, and affects the heart.

Source: Astringent taste is found in legumes such as beans and chickpeas; fruits including cranberries, pomegranates, unripe banana, pears and dried fruit; vegetables such as broccoli, okra, cauliflower, asparagus and turnip; grains such as rye, buckwheat, and quinoa; spices and herbs including turmeric and marjoram; coffee and tea. Most raw vegetables and also the skins of fruits have astringent qualities.

JNANENDRIYA: Experiencing Food Through the Senses

Besides hunger, we choose food for many reasons—personal taste, family preferences, cultural influences, emotional reasons, health concerns, societal pressures, convenience, cost, and variety and quantity of the available offerings.

The main reason why we choose to eat a particular food is that we love the taste of that food or it can be our favourite food. But sometimes wanting to eat a particular food also depends on the organoleptic properties of the food. These properties can impact our choice of food.

Organoleptic properties are the aspects of food, water, or other substances that make an individual experience via the senses—including taste, sight, smell, and touch. Organoleptic properties of food, raw food, cosmetics, etc. have a determining effect on consumption.

The physical and chemical characteristics of food are stimuli for the eye, skin, nose, and mouth whose receptors initiate impulses that travel to the brain where perception occurs. Perception or correlation of sensory impressions determines whether a dish will be accepted or rejected.

Allergic and spoiled food can be anticipated from sensory experiences. Organoleptic procedures are performed to detect disease or contamination.

Organoleptic properties of food are described as:

1) Taste (Rasa)
2) Odour (Gandha)
3) Colour
4) Texture

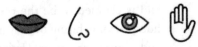

1) Taste

The sense of taste is mediated by taste receptors situated on the upper portion of the tongue and also, to a lesser extent, on the palate, pharynx, and tonsils. The receptors are said to send four different types of taste sensations to the brain and mind. The taste sensations are scattered mainly over the surface of the tongue.

The tip of the tongue is sensitive to four modalities—sweet, bitter, sour, and salty—but mainly to the sweet taste. The sides of the tongue are sensitive mainly to sour things but also to salt. The back of the tongue is sensitive to bitter foods. The taste we experience may be a result of the mixture of these primary tastes and various smells.

The sensation of hot, cold, and pain is also sent from the tongue to the brain and these play an important role in the evaluation of taste.

The nutritive power of food depends to a great extent on taste. The classification of taste is as follows:

- Sweet taste increases energy in the body and stimulates the senses. It produces moisture, cold, and heaviness. It can therefore be said to increase the tamas guna.
- Saline helps digestion, removes excess wind (vata), secretes phlegm (kapha), and is moist and warm.
- Bitter is unpalatable to the mind, but it sharpens the appetite, assists digestion, and helps eliminate toxins. It is dry, cool and light, and increases sattva guna.
- Sour is the acidic, tart taste found in vinegar, lemon, unripe fruits (sour apples, sour grapes), and products of fermentation (unsweetened yogurt or curd).

- Pungent is more an attribute of taste than a taste itself and is claimed to be the result of irritation. It is a sharp, hot, pricking, biting quality as found in chili, radish, ginger, and other such spices. Having the elements of fire and air, it is said to increase the digestive fire and the rajas guna.
- Astringent taste is dry, cool, and heavy. Lemon peel has this effect, making the mouth feel dry and contracted. It is also found in unripe fruits.

By this classification of taste, we can see that certain foods will have specific effects on the body. We can affect our temperament, body type, and so on just by the virtue of the food we eat. For example, chillies and other hot food tend to make the body more rajasic and energetic. A Sattvik or pure diet is a balanced and bland diet. When we practice yoga, diet is an adjunct to raising consciousness. Control over the senses may be a spontaneous outcome of regular yoga practice.

2) Odour

Food odours are shown to influence food choices and portion selection, and may promote a particular desire to consume certain foods. Exposure to a desirable savoury odour increases attention towards the food.

Even when satiated, the sight or smell of a desirable food can stimulate the appetite. Foot odour is a very powerful stimulus that can motivate eating in the absence of hunger, and promote positive energy balance.

The nasal apparatus is even more sensitive. We can become more conscious of its importance through meditation.

All pranayama techniques cleanse, stimulate and, eventually, awaken the sense of smell.

3) Colour

The colour of food has quite an impact on our choice of what we eat. The colour of a particular food can also influence our perception of tastes, flavours, or odours, and we often associate certain colours with particular tastes: pink with sweet things, green with salty food, and the orange and red with spicy food.

Eat Your Rainbow

Color is the single most significant product-intrinsic sensory cue when it comes to setting people's expectations regarding the likely taste and flavour of food and drink. Including different colours in your diet can ensure you're getting enough fiber, vitamins, minerals, and antioxidants, and creates a synergetic effect that helps to promote good health and lower disease risk. Most vibrantly coloured fruits and vegetables have the foremost nutrition.

For example, many red fruits and vegetables are loaded with powerful, healthy antioxidants like lycopene and anthocyanins, which fight heart conditions and prostate cancer, and decrease the danger of stroke and macular degeneration.

4) Texture

Food texture could be a collective term for sensory experiences that originate from visual, audio, and tactile stimuli. Food texture plays a vital role in influencing consumers' liking and preference for food. Among the texture characteristics, hardness/firmness is one of the most important parameters, This is often used to determine the freshness of food.

Although flavour is commonly found to be an important sensory factor responsible for the preference of food, texture is often preferred by consumers as the reason for not liking certain foods.

We generally have varying expectations of texture for different types of food. For instance, we would prefer apples to be crispy and firm, while demanding peaches and mangoes to be juicy and soft. Also, we prefer papad, khakhra, nuts and seeds to be crunchy while we like our khichdi soft.

Many different terminologies, such as firmness, juiciness, meatiness, toughness, tenderness, hardness, chewiness, stickiness, and gumminess, are used to describe various textural characteristics of different food products.

Reference

http://interscience.org.uk/v2-i2/9%20ijahm.pdf

https://www.gijhsr.com 7.pdfShadrasas (Six Types of Tastes) According To Different Ayurvedic Texts - A Literary Survey

https://www.eijo.in uploadsPDFShadrasa - Einstein International Journal Organization(EIJO)

www.yogamag.net/archives/1978/knov78/gt1178.shtml

www.yogamag.net/archives/1982/cmar82/noserose.shtml

Picture - https://swirled.com/fruits-and-vegetables-nutrients/

https://www.sciencedirect.com/topics/food-science/food-odor

https://hmhub.me/organoleptic-sensory-evaluation-product-research-development/

6

THE MIND-BODY CONNECTION

AYURVEDA AND THE GUT: BUILDING A STRONGER GUT (FODMAP)

Why is gut health given importance in Ayurveda?

Our gut is home to microflora that is composed of various species of bacteria—some harmful, some inactive and some beneficial. The good bacteria in our gut play an important role in digestion and absorption of food, preventing gut infections and maintaining immunity. The Indian medical science of Ayurveda gives immense importance to the digestive system and considers it to be the determinant of health. Moreover, other Asian medical texts, such as the Japanese *Onaka Hara* recognize the intestine as the source of spiritual and physical strength. The abdomen is regarded as the seat of the soul. Western systems of medicine have also proven that the gut microbiome is responsible for the mental health of individuals.

Symptoms of an unhealthy gut

- Irritable Bowel Syndrome (IBS)
- Blood in stools
- Flatulence
- Weight loss
- Bloating

- Poor appetite
- Regurgitation
- Abdominal cramps
- Heartburn
- Incontinence
- Nausea
- Food intolerances
- Vomiting
- Diarrhoea
- Constipation

Are you facing any digestive issues? Do you experience severe stomach cramps? Do flatulence and burping make you feel uncomfortable daily? Do you always feel bloated? If yes, then here is one of the reasons why:

Food is a collective origin of digestive symptoms. Interestingly, restricting certain food triggers can vividly improve these symptoms in sensitive people. In particular, a diet low in fermentable carbs, known as FODMAPS, has been clinically endorsed for the management of IBS.

Let's understand a FODMAP diet, how it works, and who should try it:

F: Fermentable
O: Oligosaccharides
D: Disaccharides
M: Monosaccharides
A: and P: Polyols

These are short-chain carbohydrates that resist digestion. Instead of being absorbed into the bloodstream, they reach the far end of the intestine where most of the gut bacteria use these as fuel, producing hydrogen gas, bloating, stomach cramps, pain, constipation, and diarrhea in sensitive individuals.

Why should we choose low-FODMAP foods?

1) Low FODMAP can help to reduce the risk of gas formation, bloating, diarrhea, constipation and stomach pain.
2) Low FODMAP diet may also be beneficial for people with IBS, inflammatory bowel diseases (IBD) like Crohn's disease and ulcerative colitis, and other functional gastrointestinal disorders (FGID).
3) Since digestive disturbances are also linked to stress, anxiety and depression, low FODMAP food may also cause positive psychological benefits.

Low FODMAP foods

- Meat, fish and eggs
- All fats and oils
- Most herbs and spices
- Nuts and seeds (except pistachios and cashews)
- Fruits: Bananas, blueberries, cantaloupe, grapefruit, grapes, kiwi, lemons, lime, melons (except watermelon), oranges, passion fruit, raspberries and strawberries
- Sweeteners: Maple syrup, molasses, stevia, and most sugar alcohols
- Dairy products: Lactose-free dairy products such as almond milk, rice milk and coconut milk
- Vegetables: Alfalfa, bell peppers, carrots, celery, cucumbers, eggplant, ginger, green beans, kale, lettuce, chives, olives, potatoes, radishes, spinach, spring onion (only green), squash, sweet potatoes, tomatoes, turnips, yams, water chestnuts and zucchini
- Grains: Corn, oats, rice, quinoa, sorghum (chara), tapioca
- Beverages: Water, coffee, tea, etc.

High FODMAP foods

- Excess free fructose

- Fruits: Apples, pears, mangoes, watermelons, cherries, figs
- Sweeteners and condiments: Honey, high fructose corn syrup, fruit juice concentrate
- Lactose: Milk (cow, goat, and sheep), ice cream, soft cheeses, yogurt
- Oligosaccharides
- Fruits: Watermelon, peaches
- Vegetables: Garlic, onions, shallots
- Cereals: Wheat, barley, and rye-based products (in large amounts)
- Legumes: Chickpeas, lentils, beans
- Nuts: Pistachios, cashews
- Polyols
- Fruits: Apples, apricots, pears, peaches, plums, prunes, watermelon, blackberries
- Vegetables: Cauliflower, mushrooms
- Sweeteners: Sorbitol, mannitol, maltitol, xylitol, polydextrose, isomalt

FOOD AND MOOD CONNECT

The connection between mood and food:

We already know that the food we eat plays an important role in our overall health, but did we know that it can affect our mood too? Yes, it does! It is said, 'One cannot think well, love well, sleep well if one has not dined well.' Unhealthy eating patterns can cause mood swings. Blood sugar fluctuations and nutritional imbalances are often to blame. Let's see how some unhealthy eating habits can alter the mood.

1. Skipping meals will likely leave you feeling weak and tired.
2. Reducing the variety of foods in your diet can make it more difficult to get all the essential nutrients you need. Low levels of zinc, iron, vitamin B, magnesium, vitamin D,

and omega-3 fatty acids are associated with a worsening mood and decreased energy.

3. High intakes of unhealthy, processed carbohydrates, such as white bread and pastries, cause blood sugars to rise and fall rapidly. This can lead to low energy and irritability.

Following a healthy eating plan can keep you energized and assist you to feel your best as good nutrition is a crucial component of your emotional well-being.

Here are some tips that can make you improve your eating to support your mood and your mental health:

• Eat at set intervals throughout the day and drink plenty of water.
• Choose less refined sugars and eat more wholegrains.
• Include protein in each meal and eat a variety of foods which includes omega-3 fatty acids in your diet.
• Exercise at regular intervals.

There are two types of people who eat under stress: Those who overeat and those who don't eat all. Identify yourself:

1. Do you skip most meals and hardly eat when stressed?
2. Are you a binge-eater and overeat when stressed?

Stress Eating

Stress eating entails consuming food in response to your feelings, especially when you are not hungry or don't eat anything, which can further lead to acidity, among other health issues.

Why do we eat when we are stressed?

For most of us, food offers comfort. Stress is associated with increased hunger hormones, which contribute to cravings for unhealthy foods and, unfortunately, the least healthy foods usually offer the most comfort.

How do you recognize if you're a stress-eater?

- Do you ever eat without realizing you're even doing it? Do you often feel guilty or ashamed after eating?
- After an unpleasant experience, like an argument, do you eat even when you are not feeling hungry?
- Do you eat because you feel there's nothing else to do?

How to cope up with stress eating?

There are different ways to control stress-eating and turn your stress into a more positive experience. Find the source of stress that triggers you to eat.

- If you identify your triggers, then you'll take active steps to tackle stress before it gets out of control. Once you recognize what causes you to eat more, find out healthy systems to avoid turning to food for comfort under stress. Fight your boredom and do things that calm you down, like listening to music.
- Find social support with friends and family and do the things that you would love to distract yourself from turning to food when stressed.
- One thing that sometimes does not help control stress-eating is waiting and hoping that it'll change. Take active steps today to tackle stress-eating and find new, healthy habits to manage stress.

Emotional Eating

Emotional eating affects both men and women. It may be caused by a variety of things, including stress, hormonal changes, or mixed hunger cues. It comes suddenly and one craves only for certain foods. This is not guided by the need to feel satiated, or guilt. So, one needs to be clear whether the person is hungry and eating for survival, or whether the person is an appetite-eater.

eating mindfully using the Mindful Eating Cycle learn to eat with more purpose and awareness.

5. How much do I eat?

Your stomach is only about the size of your fist, so it only takes about a palm-full of food to fill it. Through mindfulness training, you learn to determine the appropriate amount to eat by paying attention to cues and situations and overeating.

6. Where do I invest my energy?

Ask yourself: Where do I spend the fuel that is consumed? The food you consume provides the energy and nutrients to live, work, play and exercise. When you eat more than your body needs, the excess fuel will be stored to be used for fuel later. Increased physical activity in daily living will have a significant impact on your fuel balance. Doing exercise will improve your health, increase your stamina and function, and make you feel better. When you invest your energy in living a fully balanced life, you are less likely to use food to meet your needs, which would curb overeating.

What Is Mindful Yoga?

Mindfulness has always been an essential aspect of the physical practice of yoga. Mindful yoga is considered to be a form of meditation, and/or it is very often practised before a formal meditation sitting.

References: Mindful eating questionnaire in the journal of American dietetic association is developed by Celia Framson, Alan R. Kristal, Jeannette Schenk, Alyson J. Littman, Steve iadt, and Denise Benitez in 2009. Domains of the final 28-n questionnaire were: Disinhibition, Awareness, External Cues, tional Response, and Distraction

So, what are the common of causes emotional eating?

Eating your emotions can be a way to temporarily silence or stuff down uncomfortable feelings, including anger, fear, sadness, anxiety, loneliness, resentment and shame, which leads people to overeat. A person may try to compensate for feelings of unfulfillment and emptiness, and food is a way for them to occupy their mouth and time. Dining with others may be a good way to alleviate stress, but it also can lead to overeating.

How to cope with emotional eating

Dealing with negative emotions is often the first step towards overcoming emotional eating.

1. A walk, jog or a yoga routine may help in getting rid of some emotional moments.
2. Try meditation as there are a variety of studies that support mindfulness meditation as a treatment for binge-eating disorders and emotional eating.
3. Eating a healthy diet and seeking support, getting together with friends for a walk, spending time with your loved ones, and retail therapy. In other words, get involved in some activity that diverts your attention from food.
4. Food may help ease emotions initially, but addressing the feelings behind the hunger is important in the long term.
5. Also, practice mindful eating habits that may help you cope with emotional eating.

FOODS THAT KEEP STRESS AT BAY

Ways to Conquer Anxiety

Anxiety is a very common problem. It's a disorder characterized by constant worry and nervousness, and is sometimes related to poor brain health.

Foods That Can Reduce Anxiety

1. It is a herb that contains high amounts of antioxidants that helps to reduce inflammation, which might decrease the risk of anxiety.
2. **Green tea** contains L-theanine, an amino acid that has positive effects on brain health and anxiety reduction.
3. **Chia seeds** are a good source of omega-3 fatty acids, which reduces anxiety and boosts brain health.
4. **Dark chocolate** contains flavonols, which are antioxidants that benefit brain function by improving blood flow to the brain and help adapt to stressful situations.
5. **Curd** contains probiotics (healthy bacteria) that can improve several aspects of your well-being, including mental health.
6. **Almonds** provide a significant amount of antioxidants such as vitamin E, which plays a major role in anxiety prevention.
7. **Turmeric** is a spice that contains curcumin, a compound that promotes brain health and prevents anxiety disorders.

JAGRUKTA: MINDFUL EATING

What is Mindfulness?

Mindful eating means maintaining an in-the-moment awareness of the food and drink one puts into their body, observing rather than judging how the food makes one feel and the signals the body sends about taste, satisfaction and fullness. Mindful eating requires one to simply acknowledge and accept the feelings, thoughts and bodily sensations one observes—and can extend to the process of buying, preparing and serving your food as well as consuming it.

'Mindful eating is the practice of cultivating an open-minded awareness of how the food we elect to eat affects one's body, feelings, mind, and everyone who's around us. The practice

enhances our understanding of what to eat, the way to eat, what proportion to eat, and why we eat what we eat.'

The Mindful Eating Cycle

This model provides a practical but powerful structure that helps individuals identify and resolve problematic eating as well as sedentary lifestyles, regardless of size or health status. The mindful eating cycle is needed to avoid overeating and promote healthy eating. The six decisions to be made in the cycle are as follows:

1. Why do I eat?
   Many people lack an awareness and understanding of their eating choices. A person needs to ask questions like: 'Am I really hungry? Why do I think I eat? Am I aware of all the situations and/or emotions that are triggering me to want to eat when I'm not hungry?'
2. When do I feel like eating?
   This is a simple but powerful question. Whenever you feel like eating, ask yourself, 'Am I hungry?' If the answer is 'no then ask yourself why do you feel like munching. Anoth question to ask yourself is 'When do you feel like grabbi bite?' Do you reward yourself with food or do you eat to with boredom, stress, sadness, anger, loneliness and e
3. What do I eat?
   It is important to ask this question: Healthy food or this case, use balance, variety and moderation to choices. Focus on deriving the necessary nutrients. diet for nourishment with a focus on enjoyment i Consider overall dietary intake, not just the one item.
4. How do I eat?
   Many people eat quickly and/or while d activities such as watching television, d This sets the stage for overeating. Ind

MINDFUL EATING QUESTIONNAIRE

1. I eat so quickly that I don't taste what I'm eating
   a. Never/rarely
   b. Sometimes
   c. Often
   d. Usually
2. When I eat at buffets/weddings, I tend to overeat
   a. Never/rarely
   b. Sometimes
   c. Often
   d. Usually
   e. I don't eat at buffets/weddings
3. At a party or restaurant where there is a lot of good food, I notice when it makes me want to eat more food than I should
   a. Never/rarely
   b. Sometimes
   c. Often
   d. Usually/ always
4. I recognize when food advertisements make me want to eat
   a. Never/rarely
   b. Sometimes
   c. Often
   d. Usually/ always
   e. Food ads never make me want to eat
5. When a restaurant portion is too large, I stop eating when I'm full
   a. Never/rarely
   b. Sometimes
   c. Often
   d. Usually/ always

6. **My thoughts tend to wander while I am eating**
   a. Never/rarely
   b. Sometimes
   c. Often
   d. Usually/ always

7. **When I'm eating one of my favourite foods, I don't recognize when I've had enough**
   a. Never/rarely
   b. Sometimes
   c. Often
   d. Usually/ always

9. **I notice when just going into a movie theatre makes me want to eat candy or popcorn**
   a. Never/rarely
   b. Sometimes
   c. Often
   d. Usually/ always

9. **If it doesn't cost much more, I get the larger size food or drink regardless of how hungry I feel**
   a. Never/rarely
   b. Sometimes
   c. Often
   d. Usually/ always
   e. I never eat candy or popcorn

10. **I notice when there are subtle flavours in the foods I eat**
    a. Never/rarely
    b. Sometimes
    c. Often
    d. Usually/ always

11. **If there are leftovers that I like, I take a second helping even though I'm full**
    a. Never/rarely
    b. Sometimes
    c. Often

    d. Usually/ always

12. **When eating a pleasant meal, I notice if it makes me feel relaxed**
    a. Never/rarely
    b. Sometimes
    c. Often
    d. Usually/ always

13. **I snack without noticing that I am eating**
    a. Never/rarely
    b. Sometimes
    c. Often
    d. Usually/ always

14. **When I eat a big meal, I notice if it makes me feel heavy or sluggish**
    a. Never/rarely
    b. Sometimes
    c. Often
    d. Usually/ always

15. **I stop eating when I'm full even when eating something I love**
    a. Never/rarely
    b. Sometimes
    c. Often
    d. Usually/ always

16. **I appreciate the way my food looks on my plate**
    a. Never/rarely
    b. Sometimes
    c. Often
    d. Usually/ always

17. **When I'm feeling stressed at work, I'll go find something to eat**
    a. Never/rarely
    b. Sometimes
    c. Often

    d. Usually/ always

    e. I don't work

18. If there's good food at a party, I'll continue eating even after I'm full

    a. Never/rarely

    b. Sometimes

    c. Often

    d. Usually/ always

19. When I'm sad, I eat to feel better

    a. Never/rarely

    b. Sometimes

    c. Often

    d. Usually/ always

20. I notice when foods and drinks are too sweet

    a. Never/rarely

    b. Sometimes

    c. Often

    d. Usually/ always

21. Before I eat, I take a moment to appreciate the colours and smells of my food

    a. Never/rarely

    b. Sometimes

    c. Often

    d. Usually/ always

22. I taste every bite of food that I eat

    a. Never/rarely

    b. Sometimes

    c. Often

    d. Usually/ always

23. I recognize when I'm eating and not hungry

    a. Never/rarely

    b. Sometimes

    c. Often

    d. Usually/ always

e. I never eat when I'm not hungry.

24. **I notice when I'm eating from a dish of candy just because it's there**
    a. Never/rarely
    b. Sometimes
    c. Often
    d. Usually/ always

25. **When I'm at a restaurant, I can tell when the portion I've been served is too large for me**
    a. Never/rarely
    b. Sometimes
    c. Often
    d. Usually/ always

26. **I notice when the food I eat affects my emotional state**
    a. Never/rarely
    b. Sometimes
    c. Often
    d. Usually/ always

27. **I have trouble not eating ice cream, cookies, or chips if they're around the house.**
    a. Never/rarely
    b. Sometimes
    c. Often
    d. Usually/ Always

27. **I think about things I need to do while I am eating**
    a. Never/rarely
    b. Sometimes
    c. Often
    d. Usually/ always

The questions are segregated as Awareness, Distraction, Disinhibition, Emotional Response, and External Cues.

SCORE YOURSELF:

Category	Question #	Response Value	
Awareness—being aware of how food looks, tastes and smells	10		
	12		
	16		
	21		
	22		
	26		**Awareness**
	# Answered	Total	Score
Distraction—focusing on other things while eating	1		
	6		
	28		**Distraction**
	# Answered	Total	Score
Disinhibition—eating even when full	2		
	5		
	7		
	9		
	11		
	15		
	18		
	25		**Disinhibition**
	# Answered	Total	Score
Emotional Response—eating in response to sadness or stress	13		
	17*		
	19		**Emotional Response**
	27		
	# Answered	Total	Score

External Cues—eating in response to environmental cues, such as advertising	3		
	4		
	8		
	14		
	23		Emotional Cues
	24		
	# Answered	Total	Score

	Never/Rarely	4 pts.
Questions in a while shaded box	Sometimes	3 pts.
	Often	2 pts.
	Usually/Always	1 pt.
	N/A	0 pts.*
Questions in a gray shaded box	Never/Rarely	1 pt.
	Sometimes	2 pts.
	Often	3 pts.
	Usually/Always	4 pts.
	N/A	0 pts.*

CONCLUSION

The score of the above Mindful Eating Questionnaire is 1. The score must be in number between 1 and 4.

A lower score indicates a greater tendency to eat with mindfulness, while a higher score indicates that the respondent struggles to eat mindfully—or doesn't know how to eat mindfully.

What is your score? If it is not perfect or not even close to it, don't worry! Nobody is perfectly mindful all the time. Start practising the Mindful Eating Cycle, which will see you undergo a positive transformation in your life, and in your relationship to food.

✤

MOUTH FRESHENERS

Mukhwas is a colourful Indian after-meal snack or digestive aid widely used as a mouth freshener, especially after meals. It comprises various seeds and nuts, often fennel, anise, coconut, coriander, and sesame. They are sweet in flavour and highly aromatic due to added sugar. Mukhwas has various essential oils, including peppermint oil. The seeds can be savoury or sweet—coated in sugar and brightly coloured.

The word is an amalgamation of 'mukh' meaning mouth and 'was' meaning smell.

❧

THE CLASSIC FRESHENER

Total weight	350 gms
Serving size	1

Ingredients

Sesame seeds	50 gm
Fennel seeds	150 gm
Watermelon seeds	50 gm
Flax seeds	50 gm
Dhana dal	50 gm

Method

- Mix the seeds with lime juice and amchur.
- Let this rest for 10 minutes.
- Roast the sesame, fennel, and flaxseeds lightly.
- Assemble the ingredients and fill in an airtight or glass container.

❧

A FRESH SPLASH

Total weight	250 gm
Serving size	1 tsp

Ingredients

Mint leaves	60 gm
Dried rose petals	30 gm
Fennel seeds	150 gm
Cardamom seeds	10 gm

Method

- Roast the fennel and cardamom seeds lightly.
- Wrap the mint leaves in a muslin cloth and sun dry for 4-5 hours.
- Assemble all ingredients and store in an airtight or glass container.

THE FAB FIVE

Total weight	330 gm
Serving size	1

Ingredients

Basil leaves	50 gm
Fennel seeds	150 gm
Flax seeds	50 gm
Pumpkin seeds	50 gm
Onion seeds	30 gm

Method

- Roast all the seeds very lightly.

- Wrap the basil leaves in a muslin cloth and sun dry for 4-5 hours.
- Assemble all the ingredients and store in an airtight or glass jar.

❧

THE ULTIMATE DIGESTER

Total weight	280 gm
Serving size	1

Ingredients

Ajwain	75 gm
Fennel seeds	100 gm
Dhana dal	50 gm
Dry date powder	50 gm

Method

- Roast the ajwain and fennel seeds mildly.
- Powder the dried dates.
- Assemble all the ingredients and place them in an airtight or glass container.

❧

THE BOTANICAL POWER

Total weight	250 gm
Serving size	1 tsp

Ingredients

Mint leaves dried	50 gm
Basil leaves dried	50 gm
Sweetened dry rose petals	50 gm
Sunflower seeds	50 gm

Dhana dal   50 gm

Method

- Dry the mint and basil leaves by wrapping them in a muslin cloth and exposing them to sunlight for 4-5 hours.
- Grind the sunflower seeds and sweetened rose petals coarsely.
- Assemble all the ingredients in an airtight or glass jar.

❧

THE NATURAL GALACTAGOGUE

Total weight   550 gm
Serving size   1

Ingredients

Fennel seeds   200 gm
Dry coconut   100 gm
Walnuts   50 gm
Ajwain   100 gm
Sesame seeds   50 gm
Suva   50 gm

Method

- Roast the fennel seeds, ajwain, suva and sesame seeds lightly.
- Chop the walnuts coarsely and grate the dry coconut.
- Assemble all the ingredients and fill in an airtight container or glass jar.
- This is ideal for lactating mothers.

❧

KHATTA MEETHA PAAN

Serving size	2

Ingredients

Betel leaves	2 leaves
Cardamom seeds	1 tsp
Fennel seeds	2 tsp
Dhana dal	½ tsp
Rose gulkand	1 tsp
Raw mango (kachi keri)	½ tbsp
Poppy seeds (khas khas)	¼ tsp
Saffron	4-6 strands

Method

- Take a bowl, add gulkand followed by coarsely ground cardamom seeds, fennel seeds, dhana dal, and poppy seeds.
- Chop the kachi keri in juliennes.
- Later, place 1 tbsp of the gulkand mix on the betel leaf.
- Top it with chopped kachi keri and saffron strands.
- Serve the betel pan folded in a triangle and fix the fold with a toothpick if required.

7

FOOD IS DIVINITY

All living creatures of the world are born of food,
live by food and at the end they go back to become food

ANNABRAHMA: From food we come, we grow and we become

PART 1:

वदनी कवल घेता नाम घ्या श्रीहरीचे।
सहज हवन होते नाम घेता फुकाचे॥
जीवन करी जिवित्वा अन्न हे पूर्ण ब्रहम।
उदरभरण नोहे जाणिजे यज्ञकर्म॥१॥

Before consuming the first morsel of food, remember God,
Food is digested well only when you have gratitude for the same.
The food that gives us life is God itself
And the process of ingestion of food isn't mechanical but a
divine process of Oblation (Yadnya/Havan)

'Anna brahma' is translated as 'anna' i.e. food and 'Brahma' i.e. god—'food is god'.

If we consider the body to be a temple, then food becomes a kind of oblation, instead of just being something that pleases the palate.

We are what we eat, and the food we eat should also be pure and nutritious, meaning Sattvik in nature, for our well-being. The food should be regarded highly and should be clean, nutritious and fresh, providing us optimum health.

हेनजाणावेसाधारण।

अन्नबह्ममरुपजाण।

जेजीवनहेतुकारण।

विश्वायया।।

—श्रीभावार्थंदीपिका (श्री ज्ञानश्वेरी 3:33)

Saint Dnyaneshvar says, 'Food itself is Brahma.' The saying states that food should not be taken lightly, and should be regarded just as highly as God, and food is the foundation on which we are alive and the reason why our world exists.

PART 2:

Brahmārpañam Brahma Havir Brahmāgnau Brahmañāhutaṃ, Brahmaiva Tena Gantavyam Brahmakarmā Samādhinah.

The whole creation is the gross projection of Brahman, the cosmic consciousness itself; the food too is Brahman, the process of offering it is Brahman; it is being offered in the fire of Brahman. He who thus sees that Brahman is action reaches Brahman alone.

Aham Vaishvānaro Bhutvā Prāñinām Ḍehamāshritaha, Prāñāpāna Samāyuktah Pachāmyannam Chaturvidham.

I, the Supreme Spirit, abiding in the body of living beings as the Fire (Vaiswanara) in their stomach. I am associated with their Praana and Apaana, digest the four types of foods (solids, fluids, semi-fluid, and liquid) which they eat.

The two verses are from the *Bhagavad Gita*, Chapter IV, Verse 24 and Chapter XV, Verse 14, respectively.

CONNOTATION

Food that is Sattvik in nature cleanses our mind and soul, just like the properties of the food. The food offered to the Gods before eating is a form of prayer and, hence, becomes prasadam. Praying cleanses the foods that are present in the cooked form. The impurities come from the impurities present in the unclean utensils, the dirt that remains in the ingredients of the cooked food, and the unclean impurities that may be formed or ignored during the cooking process. The food must be purified for the mind to be purified too. It is not always possible to obtain the food in the best way possible since we cannot always ensure that food is cooked in a positive state of mind or we cannot always ensure if the ingredients that are sold to us were grown and handled in the best way possible. It is essential from our side to offer God the food in a form of prasadam to ensure that we always express gratitude and that the impurities that have been overlooked throughout the process may not harm us.

KRUTAGYATA: ATTITUDE AND GRATITUDE OF THE EATER

According to Ayurveda, good health comes from not only eating the right foods but also assuming the right attitude towards it. When food is eaten with a relaxed and calm mind, digestion is optimal. However, when the same food is consumed with feelings of grief, anxiety and anger, it leads to digestive ailments.

Ayurveda has recognized the intimate connection between food and the mind. Ayurvedic science transcends the qualitative and quantitative aspects of food and places profound importance on factors such as the relationship with food, the ambience in which it is cooked and consumed, and the mental attitude of the cook and recipient. To derive maximum benefit from it, there must be harmony among all the factors mentioned earlier.

Keeping this in mind, Ayurveda has recommended the

Asta 'Aahara Vidhi Vesheshayatana', or the eight guidelines for consuming food. These principles stand tall on the foundation of scientific evidence. Several modern studies now prove the relationship between our emotions and eating behaviour.

Asta Aahara Vidhi Vesheshayatana	Ishte Deshe: Always eat in a place, which is close to the kitchen. This ensures that the food served is fresh and warm. Sit comfortably and completely immerse your senses in the act of eating.
	Ishta Sarvopakaranam: Food is enjoyed to the fullest when it is accompanied by suitable accessories such as cutlery, plates, and a few accompaniments such as chutneys and salad, which make the eating experience more enjoyable.
	Nati Drutam-Nati Vilambit: This Ayurvedic principle advises against eating too quickly or too slowly. Both these behaviours may lead to digestive complaints and are indicative of stress.
	Ajalpana-Ahasana: Avoid talking or laughing while consuming food. Such behaviours may prove dangerous as they may place the food inappropriately in your body. These distractions may also result in overeating or eating unhealthy. Food must be consumed with complete attention.
	Tanmana Bhunjeet: Eating with complete awareness is one of the most important teachings of Ayurveda. Focused eating helps one to enjoy the experience thoroughly and results in healthy food choices. This behaviour also promotes individuals' mental health.

> **Atmanambhisamikshya Samyaka:** The final principle urges individuals to pick food wisely and eat according to one's prakruti (body constitution). Eat according to your body's requirement and learn to be intuitive towards your body's signals. What you crave is what your body lacks.

Spirit of Gratitude

In the Vedic age, prayers were offered to the higher powers of nature, as it is both the provider and the destroyer. To appease the forces and thank them for their constant mercy, prayers of gratitude were chanted.

BHOJANAM MANTRA

This vedic prayer invokes the universe to provide food for all beings:

Om annapate annasyano dehyanamīvasya śuṣmiṇaḥ
pra pradātāraṃ tāriṣa ūrjanno dhehi dvipade catuṣpade
(May our body get nourished by the food we consume
Bless everyone with food)

Om svādo pīto madho pīto vayaṃ
tvā vavṛmahe asmākamavītā bhava
(Bless us with good health and vitality, O provider of food)

Om moghamannam vindate apracetāḥ
satyaṃ bravīmi vadha itsatasya
nāryamaṇaṃ puṣyati no sakhāyaṃ
kevalāgho bhavati kevalādī
(One who seeks food without labour, is foolish
Food obtained thus, would only bring unhappiness
One who eats alone, would succumb to guilt

Bless us, that we share and eat always with others)

oṃ śāntiḥ śāntiḥ śāntiḥ
(Om Peace, Peace, Peace)

Annastuti (Praising food)

O sweet food, honeyed food,
we have chosen you: for us be a helper.

The verses of hymn 187 of the *Rigveda* give a charming acknowledgement to food—that which nourishes. Moreover, natural forces such as wind, rain and earth are also revered as they bring food.

8

MYTHS AND FACTS

MYTH 1: AYURVEDIC DIET AND LIFESTYLE ARE EXPENSIVE

Fact: Ayurveda always recommends using produce that is seasonal and local. These ingredients always tend to be cheaper at the local farmer's market. Moreover, most of the recipes are simple and do not require expensive cookware or staples. Ayurvedic lifestyle mostly requires you to adopt simple practices and behaviour modifications and does not expect you to invest in material goods.

MYTH 2: AYURVEDIC COOKING IS TIME-CONSUMING

Ayurvedic cooking usually does not involve elaborate steps and complicated techniques. The preparation time is minimal in Ayurvedic cooking since it urges people to eat fresh. Pre-soaking your grains and pulses brings down the cooking time significantly.

MYTH 3: AYURVEDIC PRINCIPLES ARE ANCIENT AND OUTDATED

Ayurveda is timeless wisdom that promotes the holistic nature of health. Most of the dietary principles and health guidelines take us back to the core concepts of Ayurveda. They are as relevant today, as they were several years back.

MYTH 4: AYURVEDIC REMEDIES TAKE TIME TO SHOW RESULTS

While dealing with health, patience and consistency are key. Furthermore, the herbs and medicinal formulations advocated by Ayurveda are powerful and must be consumed only after consulting a professional doctor.

MYTH 5: AYURVEDA AND WESTERN MEDICINE ARE AT LOGGERHEADS

Many recent studies and investigations have proven that Ayurveda has a very strong scientific foundation. Western medicine has also acknowledged Ayurveda's effectiveness and approved its principles.

UPAVASA OR FASTING

Upavasa or fasting remains an important component of festivals and cultural ceremonies in India. A few people set aside auspicious days in their annual calendars to observe fasts. Ayurvedic medical texts have defined fasting as the abstinence from chewing, licking, swallowing and drinking. Fasting is an integral part of the Ayurvedic detoxification therapy called Panchakarma. Ayurvedic texts have mentioned numerous therapeutic benefits of fasting for various diseases.

Benefits of Fasting:

- It kindles Agni, the digestive fire.
- In the case of mild fever, fasting is beneficial.
- It prevents the accumulation of toxins in the channels of the body.
- Acharya Dalhana has recommended that in case of eye disorders such as conjunctivitis, one must fast for three days

or consume food only during the night.

- Fasting is an effective management trick for diarrhea and vomiting. It regulates the digestion process and helps the individual regain strength.
- Fasting has preventive effects against cancer and other metabolism-related disorders.
- Studies have shown that women with polycystic ovary syndrome (PCOS) have benefitted from fasting. Short episodes of calorie restrictions improve psychological health, regulate the menstrual cycle, and boost women's reproductive health.
- Fasting stimulates parathyroid hormone secretion, which is good for your bone health.
- Research shows that planned fasting for just four weeks can reduce weight, body mass index and waist circumference. It, therefore, helps in controlling metabolic disorders.
- Fasting positively affects mental health. It improves self-esteem and reduces feelings of anxiety and depression.

Here's how you must feel when you observe a fast:

- Lightness and freshness in the body
- Regular and normal elimination of urine, flatus and stool
- Reduced drowsiness and lethargy
- Improved appetite
- A calm mind

Extended periods of fasting must be performed under expert guidance. In case you observe the following symptoms, you are going wrong with your fasting practice:

- Excessive saliva production.
- Loss of taste, impaired hearing and problems with vision
- Cracking joints
- Tiredness and apathy
- Cough
- Loss of appetite

- Dryness of mouth and excessive thirst
- Increased belching

It is suggested that fasting must be followed by consuming a freshly cooked meal of rice gruel that is easy to digest and a good appetizer.

The classical texts of Ayurveda have advised against fasting for the following conditions:

- Individuals with diseases due to elevated vata
- Hernia
- Those who have very strong hunger and thirst pangs
- Undernourished, old or very young individuals
- Pregnant women
- Individuals suffering from psychological extremities such as extreme rage or jealousy.

REFERENCES

CHAPTER 1

Ayurveda: Historical, Philosophical, Conceptual and Sustainable Perspectives - shodhganga.inflibnet.ac.in
Ayurvedic Concept of Food and Nutrition by Amala Guha
Ayurvedic Science of Food and Nutrition by Sanjeev Rastogi
Dietetics in Ayurveda: The forgotten science, ijrap.net; Dua Pradeep and Dua Pamila
Effect of yogic practices with yogic diet on selected biochemical variables among stressed housewives, *International Journal of Yogic, Human Movement and Sports Sciences* 2018; 3 (2): 941-942
Dua Pradeep et al/ IJRAP 2011, 2 (4) 1005-1010
Evidence-based practice in complementary and alternative medicine: Sanjeev Rastogi
Finding your dosha (life force) review by Jonathan Collin, MD
Food as a link between the visible and the invisible: an exploration into Hindu rituals: *The Investigator*, an international peer-reviewed journal of multidisciplinary explorations, Vol. 02, No. 2, June 2016
Effect of yogic practices on nutritional and academic performance of the selected adolescents, P. Nazni, J. Bhuvaneswari, and Ravinder Singh; *Official Journal of IIFAN*
International J. of Healthcare and Biomedical Research, Volume: 05, Issue: 02, January 2017, 59-71
Complete Book of Ayurveda by Hans H. Rhyner
Hatha Yoga Pradipika by Swami Swatmaram Swami Muktibodhananda
International Journal of Innovative Research and Advanced Studies (IJIRAS) Volume 06, Issue 10, October 2019
Dube, K. C., Kumar, A., & Dube, S. (1983). *Personality Types in Ayurveda*. *The American Journal of Chinese Medicine, 11 (01n04)*, 25–34.
South Asia: Journal of South Asian Studies, n.s., Vol. XXXI, No. 1, April 2008
Chandogya Upanishad translated by Max Mueller The Bhagavad Gita

'Food in the Vedic Tradition', Author(s): Dina Simoes Guha, Source: *India International Centre Quarterly*, Vol. 12, No. 2, FOOD CULTURE (JUNE 1985), pp. 141-152

'Linkage of concepts of good nutrition in yoga and modern science', Author(s): Vaishali V. Agte and Shashi A. Chiplonkar, Source: *Current Science*, Vol. 92, No. 7 (10 April 2007), pp. 956-961

The Investigator: An International Refereed Journal of Multidisciplinary Explorations (Vol. 2, No. 2) June 2016

Indian Journal of Dermatology, Venereology and Leprology, 01 Jan 1980, 46(1):23-27

PMID: 28218086

Indian food and cuisine: A historical survey by Rekha Pande

Chapter 2

Ayu, 2010 Jul–Sep; 31(3): 395–398

Divya et al., AlternInteg Med 2013, 2:8

Ayurveda (Idiot's guides) by Sahara Rose Ketabi

Theyogainstitute.org

Vol. 2, Issue-01, ISSN: 2456-82799 Sujitkumar et at. JIF: 1.021

Int. J. Pharm. Med. Res. 2015; 3(1):186–190

Global J. Res. Med. Plants & Indigen. Med. | Volume 2, Issue 5 | May 2013 | 380–385

Chapter 6

https://www.mentalhealthfirstaid.org/external/2018/03/relationship-food-mood

https://www.mayoclinic.org/healthy-lifestyle/weight-loss/in-depth/weight-loss/art-20047342

Adapted from shared resources at Fred Hutchinson Cancer Center (http://sharedresources.fhcrc.org/). Based on Framson C, Kristal AR, Schenk JM, Littman AJ, Zeliadt S, Benitez D. Development and validation of the Mindful Eating Questionnaire. J Am Diet Assoc. 2009; 109:1439-1444

Chapter 7

Rastogi S. (2014) *Applying Ayurvedic Eating Principles to the Science of Stress-Linked Food Behavior.* In: Rastogi S. (eds) Ayurvedic Science of Food and Nutrition. Springer, New York, NY

GLOSSARY

CEREALS
White rice	*Chaval*
Barley	*Jau*
Black rice	
Broken wheat	*Dalia*
Brown rice	*Bhura chaval*
Multigrain bread	
Oats	
Quinoa	
Samo rice	
Semolina	*Rava*
Sorghum	*Jowar*
Soybean	
Tapioca/Sago	*Sabudana*
Wheat	*Gehu*
White bread	
Whole wheat bread	

MILLETS
Barnyard millet	*Samvat chaval*
Buckwheat	*Kuttu*
Finger millet	*Ragi*
Foxtail millets	*Kangni*
Kodo millet	*Varagu*
Pearl millet	*Bajra*

PULSE
Bengal gram	*Herbera/Black chana*
Black chana	Kala chana
Black gram	*Udad Dal*
Chickpea	*Chhole*
Green gram	*Mung*

Mung dal *yellow*	*Mung Dal*
Pigeon pea	*Arhar/Tur Dal*
Red kidney beans	*Rajma*
Split red gram	*Masoor Dal*
Yellow mung dal	

MILK AND MILK PRODUCT

Buffalo milk	*Bhains Ka Doodh*
Buttermilk	*Chaas*
Cheese	
Cow milk paneer	
Cow's milk	*Gai Ka Doodh*
Curd	*Dahi*

PROTEIN RICH

Soya chunk
Soya milk
Tofu

VEGETABLES

Bell pepper	*Shimla Mirch*
Bitter gourd	*Karela*
Bottle gourd	*Lauki*
Brinjal/ Aubergine	*Baingan*
Broad beans	
Broccoli	
Cabbage	*Patta Gobhi*
Cauliflower	*Ful Gobhi*
Cherry tomatoes	
Cluster beans	*Guar*
Cucumber	*Kakdi/Kheera*
Drumstick	*Sahjan/Moringa*
Green peas	*Hara vatana*
Gunda	
Pointed gourd	*Parwal*
Pumpkin	*Kaddu*
Purple cabbage	
Ridge gourd	*Ghosale Ghire*
Snake gourd	*Chichinda*
Spiny gourd	Kantola

Tomato	*Tamattar*
Water chestnut	*Singhaada*
Zucchini	

GREEN LEAFY VEGETABLES

Amaranth	*Cholai*
Bathua	
Betel	*Paan*
Colocasia	*Arbi*
Coriander	*Dhanya*
Fenugreek leaves	*Methi*
Drumstick	*Moringa*
Celery	
Curry leaves	*Kadi patta*
Kale	
Lettuce	
Mint	*Pudhina*
Mustard	*Rai*
Parsley	
Radish leaves	*Muli*
Dill leaves	*Shepu*

ROOTS AND TUBERS

Onion	*Kanda, pyaaz*
Beetroot	*Beet, chukandar*
Ginger	*Adrak*
Potato	*Aloo*
Radish	*Muli*
Carrot	*Gajar*
Sweet potato	*Shakarkand*
Turnip	*Shalajam*
Celery root	*Celeriac*

FRUITS

Apple	*Safarchand*
Apricot	*Khubani*
Avocado	
Bael fruit	
Banana	*Kela*
Cherry	

Chickoo	*Sapota*
Coconut	*Narial*
Cranberry	*Karonda*
Custard apple	*Sitafal*
Fig	*Anjeer*
Grapes	*Angoor*
Guava	*Peru*
Jackfruit	*Fanas*
Kiwi	
Lemon	*Nimbu*
Lychee	
Mango	*Aam*
Muskmelon	*Kharbooja*
Orange	*Santara*
Papaya	*Papeeta*
Peach	*Aadoo*
Pear	*Naashapaatee*
Pineapple	*Ananas*
Plum	*Alubukhara*
Pomegranate	*Anaar*
Raw mango	*Kaccha aam*
Raw papaya	*Kaccha papeeta*
Strawberry	
Sweet corn	*Bhutta*
Sweet lime	*Mosambi*
Tomato	*Tamatar*
Watermelon	*Tarabooj*

BERRIES

Amla	*Gooseberry*
Blueberry	
Cranberry	
Indian jujube/ Indian Ber or Bor	
Mulberry	*Shahtut*
Raspberry	
Strawberry	
Tomato	

DRY FRUITS

Dry coconut	*Sukha Narial*

Dry fig	*Anjeer*
Prunes	*Sukha Alubukhara*

NUTS

Almonds	*Badam*
Cashew nut	*Kaju*
Dates	*Khajur*
Dry fig	*Anjeer*
Peanut	*Mungfali*
Pine nuts	*Chilgoza*
Pistachio	*Pista*
Walnuts	*Akharot*

SEEDS

Basil seeds	*Tulsi beej*
Black sesame seeds	*Kale til*
Chia seeds	
Fennel seeds	*Saunf*
Flaxseed	*Alashi*
Garden cress seeds	*Halim ke Beej*
Melon seeds	*Sakarteti ke beej*
Pumpkin seeds	*Kaddu ke Beej*
Sesame seeds	*Til*
Sunflower seeds	*Surajmukhi ke Beej*
Watermelon seeds	*Tarbuj ke Beej*

FLOWERS

Banana flower	*Kelphul*
Chamomile	*Babuna*
Hibiscus flower	*Jasvand*
Jasmine flowers	*Mogra*
Lavender	*Ustukhududs*
Meadowsweet	
Passion flower	*Krishna Kamal*
Primerose	*Basanti gulab*
Rosemary	
Roses	*Gulab*

OILS

Butter	*Makkhan*

Coconut oil	*Nariyal Ka Tel*
Cow's ghee	*Gaay Ka Ghee*
Cream	*Malaee*
Groundnut oil	*Singdana/Mungfali Ka Tel*
Khoya	*Mawa*
Mustard oil	*Sarso Ka Tel*
Olive oil	*Jetun Ka Tel*
Rice bran oil	*Chaawal Ki Bhusi Ka Tel*
Sesame oil	*Til Ka Tel*
Soybean oil	*Soya Ka Tel*
Sunflower oil	*Surajmukhi Ka Tel*

SUGARS

Black sugar	
Brown sugar	*Bhura shakkar*
Fruit jam	
Fruit squash	
Honey	*shahad*
Icing sugar	
Jaggery	*Gudd*
Maple syrup	
Misri sugar	*Khadi shakkar*
White granulated sugar	*shakkar*

FUNCTIONAL FOODS

Chikoo	*Sapota*
Fenugreek seeds	*Methi beej*
Garlic	*Lahsun*
Turmeric	*Haldi*
Wheat grass	*Gehu ki Ghaas*

SALT

Black salt	*Kala Namak*
Epsom salt	
Monosodium glutamate	*MSG*
Pink salt	*Himalayan Salt*
Rock salt (Sendha Namak)	
Sodium benzoate	
Sodium bicarbonate	
Sodium chloride	*Namak*

Sodium hydroxide

TRADITIONAL SPICES

Amchur powder	*Dry mango powder*
Asafoetida	*Hing*
Ashwagandha	
Bay leaf	*Tej patta*
Cardamom	*Elaichi*
Carrom seeds	*Ajwain*
Cinnamon	*Dalchini*
Cloves	*Laung*
Coriander seeds	*Dhaniya*
Cumin seeds	*Jeera*
Dried kokam	*Amsul*
Fennel seeds	*Saunf*
Fenugreek seeds	*Methi*
Ginger	*Adrakh*
Long pepper	*Pipali*
Mace	*Jaipatri*
Mandukaparni	*Brahmi*
Mustard seeds	*Rai*
Nutmeg	*Jaiphal*
Onion seeds	*Kalonji*
Oregano	
Pepper	*Miri*
Saffron	*Kesar*
Star anise	*Chakra phool*
Triphala	
Turmeric	*Haldi*

MEDICINAL LEAVES

Carom leaf	*Ajwain/Ova*
Holy-Basil leaf	*Tulsi ka patta*
Mango leaf	*Aam ka patta*
Neem leaf	
Papaya leaf	*Papeete ka Patta*
Plantain leaf	*Kele ka patta*
Pumpkin leaf	*Ugu*
Tamarind leaf	*Imli ka patta*
Watercress leaf	*Haleem ka patta*

ALTERNATIVE MILK
Coconut milk   *Narial ka dudh*
Almond milk   *Badam ka dudh*
Cashew milk   *Kaju ka dudh*
Hemp milk
Macademia milk
Oat milk
Quinoa milk
Soy milk

INDEX OF RECIPES

Snacks

Upma/Dalia

Uttapam

Vegetable Snacks

Steamed Snacks

Appam

Dhokla

Mouth Fresheners